M000267994

" 'There are weeks when decades ha
revolution. More than a century latei
today's finest thinkers, reports from w
crisis, speaking with urgency and fierce
plague if you wish to ignore our funda........ precariousness. Bristling with
electric truth, this collection will offer another chance, new antibodies, a
biobank for the future."

– **Patricia Gherovici**, psychoanalyst and author of
Transgender Psychoanalysis

"The impossible has happened! Capitalism has been brought to heel by the
force of a pandemic. What new thought does the virus make possible? What has
the pandemic touched in all of us? As the philosopher Jean-Luc Nancy reflects:
'Does this mean we are in a better position to reflect on this community?
The problem is that the virus is still its main representative; that between the
surveillance model and the welfare model, only the virus remains as a common
property.' And yet, this collection of essays testifies to beginning to think
together at the place of the virus, showing how it exposes the imbrication of
politics and life, and the ever present denial of death that guides our violent
compulsion to repeat. In a moment where life and death are being weighed
anew, we need these public intellectuals more than ever."

– **Jamieson Webster, Ph.D.**, psychoanalyst, author,
professor at The New School

"Coronavirus has occasioned an outpouring of theoretical speculation. It has
produced intellectual whiplash as it prompts conservatives to sound like leftists
and leftists to echo conservative talking points. Here is a collection that will
allow us to keep track of where everyone stands. *Coronavirus, Psychoanalysis, and
Philosophy* collects work from our most important theorists on the outbreak and
puts them in dialogue with each other and with the most important thinkers
from the past. The result is an absolute necessity for anyone hoping to gain a
sense of where we stand today."

– **Todd McGowan, Ph.D.**, author and professor
at University of Vermont

"Covid-19 has undoubtedly been the phenomenon of our time – in the true
sense of the phenomenal; it figures uniquely for all who encounter it and what
we encounter when we encounter it is never a thing in itself, but is always
overdetermined through the lens of science, of the social, the political, the
medical, the conspiratorial. This exceptional collection of interactive essays
captures this phenomenal moment in all its complexity, opening up the key
question, which is not, what is covid-19? but is rather, what do we do with the
multifaceted experience that is covid-19?"

– **Dr Calum Neill**, associate professor of psychoanalysis and cultural
theory at Edinburgh Napier University

Coronavirus, Psychoanalysis, and Philosophy

Originally published in the *European Journal of Psychoanalysis* (*EJP*), the essays in this volume are a set of responses to the coronavirus crisis by distinguished philosophers and psychoanalysts from around the globe.

The coronavirus irrupted, making swift and deep cuts in the fabric of our existence: the risks of contagion and indefinite periods of isolation have radically altered the functioning of society. Pandemics do not wait for comprehension in order to proliferate. Confusion, sickness, and death punctuate the failure of governments worldwide to respond. This collection of writings examines the effects of the pandemic and the conditions that make possible such a global crisis. The writers provoke us to consider how capitalism, governmental power, and biopolitics mold the contours of life and death. The contributors in this collection ignite urgent political dialogue, address emergent transformations in the social field, and offer perspectives on shifts in subjectivity and psychoanalytic practice. Beyond providing reflections on the impact of the coronavirus, the authors point to determinants of how the crisis will unfold and what may be on the horizon.

This book will be invaluable to psychoanalysts, psychotherapists, philosophers, and to all of those interested in the implications of the virus for psychoanalytic practice and theory and the social, cultural and political spheres of our world.

Fernando Castrillón, Psy.D., Editor in Chief of the *European Journal of Psychoanalysis*, is a personal and supervising psychoanalyst, professor in the Community Mental Health Program at the California Institute of Integral Studies (CIIS), and a member of the Istituto Elvio Fachinelli ISAP (Institute of Advanced Studies in Psychoanalysis) based in Rome, Italy. He is the author of a book and numerous articles in both Spanish and English.

Thomas Marchevsky, Ph.D., is an editor of the *European Journal of Psychoanalysis* and has a psychoanalytic practice in San Francisco, California. He is Clinical Director of The Clinic Without Walls and an adjunct faculty member at the California Institute of Integral Studies (CIIS).

Coronavirus, Psychoanalysis, and Philosophy

Conversations on Pandemics, Politics, and Society

Edited by Fernando Castrillón and Thomas Marchevsky

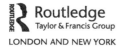

Routledge
Taylor & Francis Group

LONDON AND NEW YORK

First published 2021
by Routledge
2 Park Square, Milton Park, Abingdon, Oxon OX14 4RN

and by Routledge
52 Vanderbilt Avenue, New York, NY 10017

Routledge is an imprint of the Taylor & Francis Group, an informa business

British Library Cataloguing-in-Publication Data
A catalogue record for this book is available from the British Library

Library of Congress Cataloging-in-Publication Data
Names: Castrillón, Fernando, editor. | Marchevsky, Thomas, 1981– editor.
Title: Coronavirus, psychoanalysis, and philosophy : conversations on pandemics, politics, and society / edited by Fernando Castrillón and Thomas Marchevsky.
Description: Milton Park, Abingdon, Oxon ; New York, NY : Routledge, 2021. | Includes bibliographical references and index.
Identifiers: LCCN 2020046939 (print) | LCCN 2020046940 (ebook) | ISBN 9780367713645 (hardback) | ISBN 9780367713669 (paperback) | ISBN 9781003150497 (ebook)
Subjects: LCSH: COVID-19 (Disease) | COVID-19 (Disease)— Philosophy. | COVID-19 (Disease)—Political aspects. | COVID-19 (Disease)—Social aspects.
Classification: LCC RA644.C67 C683 2021 (print) | LCC RA644.C67 (ebook) | DDC 614.5/92414—dc23
LC record available at https://lccn.loc.gov/2020046939
LC ebook record available at https://lccn.loc.gov/2020046940

ISBN: 978-0-367-71364-5 (hbk)
ISBN: 978-0-367-71366-9 (pbk)
ISBN: 978-1-003-15049-7 (ebk)

Typeset in Bembo
by Apex CoVantage, LLC

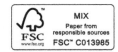

MIX
Paper from
responsible sources
FSC® C013985
www.fsc.org

Printed in the United Kingdom
by Henry Ling Limited

To the memory of the following women: Leonor Quintero Castrillón, Leonor Hurtado Echeverri, Cupertina Castrillón Mendoza, Kim Johnson Bogart, and Audrey Albrecht. A tribute to each of you lives on in me.

—Fernando Castrillón

For Chögyal Namkhai Norbu and Roger B. Levin

—Thomas Marchevsky

Contents

Contributors

Zsuzsa Baross is the author of *Posthumously, for Jacques Derrida* (2010); *Encounters: Gérard Titus-Carmel, Jean-Luc Nancy, Claire Denis* (2015); *On Contemporaneity, after Agamben, Vol. I* (2020); and *Art in the Time that Remains Vol. II* (forthcoming). Her other writings on art, temporality, and the political appeared in anthologies and journals.

Sergio Benvenuto, psychoanalyst and philosopher, is First Researcher at the Italian Council for Scientific Research. Founder and co-editor of the *European Journal of Psychoanalysis*, he has published *Conversations with Lacan* (2020).

Néstor Braunstein is an MD, psychiatrist, and psychoanalyst. He was a postgraduate professor until 2013 (México, UNAM). He is author of 25 books and hundreds of articles in different languages. His most well known book is *Jouissance. A Lacanian Concept* (2020), original in Spanish (1990 and 2006).

Massimo De Carolis is Full Professor of Political Philosophy and Social Philosophy at the University of Salerno, where he is the head of the Laboratory of Research on Human Nature and Society. Among his most recent books are *La vita nell'epoca della sua riproducibilità tecnica* (2004); *Nuovi disagi nella civiltà* (written in collaboration with Francesca Borrelli, Francesco Napolitano, and Massimo Recalcati, 2013); *Il rovescio della libertà* (2017); and *The Anthropological Paradox* (2018).

Fernando Castrillón is a personal and supervising psychoanalyst, faculty of the Psychoanalytic Institute of Northern California (PINC), a licensed clinical psychologist, Full Professor in the Community Mental Health Program at the California Institute of Integral Studies (CIIS), and the founder of the Foundation of California Psychoanalysis (FCP). He is the Editor in Chief of the *European Journal of Psychoanalysis*; a member of the Istituto Elvio Fachinelli ISAP (Institute of Advanced Studies in Psychoanalysis) based in Rome, Italy; and serves on the board of directors of the Berkeley Psychoanalytic Society (BPS). He has published a book and numerous articles in both Spanish and English and is currently writing a multivolume work on psychoanalysis, the discourse of capitalism, and the California Dream.

Divya Dwivedi is a philosopher based in the subcontinent. She teaches philosophy and literature at the Department of Humanities and Social Sciences, Indian Institute of Technology Delhi. She is the co-author with Shaj Mohan of *Gandhi and Philosophy: On Theological Anti-Politics* (2019).

Roberto Esposito, born in Italy, teaches theoretical philosophy at the Scuola Normale Superiore. Among his books, translated into numerous languages, are *Communitas. The Origin and Destiny of Community* (2004); *Immunitas: The Protection and Negation of Life* (2011); *Bios. Biopolitics and Philosophy* (Minnesota, 2008); *Third Person. Politics of Life and Philosophy of the Impersonal* (2012); *Living Thought. The Origin and Actuality of Italian Philosophy* (2012); *Two. The Machine of Political Philosophy and the Place of Thought* (2015); *Persons and Things. From the Body's Point of View* (2015); *Politics and Negation. For an Affirmative Philosophy* (2019); *A Philosophy of Europe. From the Outside* (2018); and *Instituting Thought* (2020).

Julia Kristeva is a writer, psychoanalyst, and Professor Emeritus at the University of Paris Diderot-Paris 7. She is a tutelary member of the Psychoanalytical Society of Paris and the first laureate of the Holberg Prize in December 2004. She was awarded the Hannah Arendt Prize in December 2006 and the Vaclav Havel Prize in 2008. In 2008 she created the Prize Simone de Beauvoir for the freedom of women.

Monique Lauret is a psychiatrist, psychoanalyst, and member of the Société de Psychanalyse Freudienne (SPF) and of the European Foundation for Psychoanalysis. She is the author of *L'énigme de la pulsion de mort – Pour une éthique de la joie* (2014) and *Lectures du rêve* (2011).

René Lew is a psychoanalyst practicing in Paris. He is the medical director of a community child and adolescent mental health clinic (Ivry-sur-Seine) and an attending psychiatrist at the Hôpital Esquirol. He is a co-founder and member of Dimensions de la Psychanalyse and the executive editor of the journal *Cahiers de lectures freudiennes*, as well as the founder and president of La Lysimage, an association dedicated to psychoanalytic formation, publishing, and outreach. The author of many articles on psychoanalysis, he is currently focusing on clinical work with autistic and psychotic children.

Thomas Marchevsky, Ph.D., has a psychoanalytic practice in San Francisco is a clinical supervisor, and an editor of the *European Journal of Psychoanalysis*. He is Clinical Director of the Clinic Without Walls and an adjunct faculty member at the California Institute of Integral Studies.

Shaj Mohan is a philosopher based in the subcontinent. He is the co-author with Divya Dwivedi of *Gandhi and Philosophy: On Theological Anti-Politics* (2019). His research and publications are in the areas of philosophy of technology, metaphysics, reason, politics, and truthness.

Jean-Luc Nancy teaches philosophy at the University of Strasbourg and previously taught at the University of California, San Diego. Among his works are *Le titre de la lettre. Une lecture de Lacan* (1972) and *L'Absolu littéraire* (1978) (both with Philippe Lacoue-Labarthe); *La communauté désoeuvrée* (1986, 2001); *L'expérience de la liberté* (1988); *Etre singulier pluriel* (1996); *Hegel, L'inquiétude du négatif* (1997); *Le regard du portrait* (2000); *L'il y a du rapport sexuel* (2001).

Dany Nobus is Professor of Psychoanalytic Psychology at Brunel University London, Founding Scholar of the British Psychoanalytic Society, and former chair and fellow of the Freud Museum London. He has published numerous books and papers on the history, theory, and practice of psychoanalysis, the history of psychiatry, and the history of ideas.

Rocco Ronchi is professor of theoretical philosophy at the University of L'Aquila. He teaches philosophy at Research Institute of Applied Psychoanalysis (IRPA) in Milan. Among his most recent publications are *Come fare. Per una resistenza filosofica* (2012); *Gilles Deleuze* (2015); *Il canone minore. Verso una filosofia della natura* (2017 [French translation: *La Ligne Mineure. Pour une philosophie de la nature* (2019)]); *Bertolt Brecht* (2017).

Duane Rousselle, PhD, is an associate professor and coordinator of the psychology and sociology programs in the Faculty of Liberal Arts at NMIMS, Mumbai. He is also a Lacanian psychoanalyst. His recent books include *Lacan Realism: Political and Clinical Psychoanalysis* (2017); *Gender, Sexuality & Subjectivity: A Lacanian Exploration of Language, Identity & Queer Theory* (Routledge); and *Jacques Lacan & American Sociology* (2020).

Elettra Stimilli is Professor in the Department of Philosophy at the Sapienza University of Rome. She authored numerous essays that revolve around the relationship between politics and religion, focusing particularly on contemporary thought. Among others are "The Debt of the Living" (2017) and "Debt and Guilt" (2018).

Miguel Vatter teaches politics and philosophy at Flinders University, Australia. His main research areas are republicanism, biopolitics, and political theology. Among his recent books are *The Republic of the Living. Biopolitics and the Critique of Civil Society* (2014) and *Divine Democracy. Political Theology After Carl Schmitt* (forthcoming).

Permissions

Acknowledgements

Fernando Castrillón: I extend my profound gratitude to my trusted friend, co-editor, and fellow traveler Thomas Marchevsky for his superb and diligent work on this volume. Our respective orbits have intersected for many years now and I am appreciative of the numerous and varied gifts he has brought to bear in my life. It was my dear friend Kaisa Puhakka that first suggested that we meet. Thomas and I have been laboring together on one project or another since that auspicious initial encounter. I am deeply grateful to be able to count on him as a thinker, co-conspirator, and fellow clinician. Our work on this volume has brought a host of rewards in its wake, not least of which is the reminder that the combination of creative work and friendship is one of the great and sustaining joys of life.

I offer a special note of gratitude and appreciation to my cherished friend and collaborator Sergio Benvenuto. I first met Sergio seven years ago on a trip to Rome. We came to know each other over a dinner of local delicacies in Trastevere. Our similar and heterodox sensibilities quickly brought us to work together. Our collective editorial efforts at the *European Journal of Psychoanalysis* (*EJP*) have produced equal measures of creativity, meaning, laughter, and enlightenment. It is an honor to be able to extend his editorial legacy into the future. It is important to note that it was Sergio who first introduced the idea not only of starting the coronavirus "Tribunes" in the pages of the journal but also of collecting the coronavirus essays from the *EJP* into a book. As catalyst for and assembler of the following essays, his efforts mark every page of this volume.

Two other *EJP* colleagues deserve special mention. Fellow *EJP* core editor Pietro Pascarelli has been an indispensable part of the journal. His attention to detail and literary sensibilities were crucial ingredients during our review of the coronavirus submissions to the journal. Among other things, we bonded over our common appreciation of Carlo Levi's work. I prize our growing friendship and look forward to further engagement in the future.

This volume and the journal more generally have benefitted enormously from the diligence, intelligence, and wit of managing editor Stephen Mosblech. Stephen threw himself into the work of this book from the very beginning and his hidden imprint is found throughout. His copy-editing skills, deep artistic acumen, and subtle reminders regarding the many small details of an endeavor of this sort have made the book possible. As editor of the journal, I rely on Stephen's ample capacities on a daily basis; the *EJP*'s smooth functioning is due in large part to his abiding and gifted labors. For all that and more, he has my gratitude. As well, I would like to thank the California Institute of Integral Studies (CIIS) for their generous funding of the managing editor position for the journal.

The success of any journal is built on the unstinting support and labor of its editorial board. A heartfelt note of appreciation goes out to the following individuals: Benjamin Davidson, Ed Pluth, Christopher Chamberlin, Danella Biondini, Marcus Coelen, Victor Mazin, Hannes Nykänen, Matthew Oyer, Svetlana Uvarova, Cristiana Cimino, and Claudia Vaughn. The ongoing vitality of the journal also owes its existence to the generous work of its peer reviewers and collaborators. While they are too numerous to name individually, I warmly acknowledge their ongoing support of and engagement with the journal.

I am particularly grateful to the contributors to this volume. Their submissions have left an indelible mark on my sensibilities and outlook. I thank each of them for their courage, engagement, and sincerity.

The French have captured something of the essence with their proverb, "Gratitude is the memory of the heart," which is helpful in that an expression of appreciation such as this acknowledgment is always a vexed and daunting task. There is absolutely no way I can include everyone that I would like to (my sincere apologies to those I have neglected to mention), nor can I fully express the sense of debt that I carry with me and which forms part of the basis for our common tie. Debt in this sense is generative and unfolding, allowing friendship and camaraderie to grow and flourish. In line with this, I would like to extend my heartfelt gratitude to the following individuals: Néstor Braunstein, Jamieson Webster, Patricia Gherovici, Margot Beattie and the good folks at the Berkeley Psychoanalytic Society, Bruce Fink, Domenico Cosenza, Daniel Koren, Norberto Ferrer, Dany Nobus, Annie Rogers, Beatrice Patsalides Hofmann, Bret Fimiani, Cécile Gouffrant McKenna, Christopher Meyer, Jon Bathori, Marcelo Estrada, Roberto Lazcano, Stephanie Swales, Nathan Lupo, Diana Cuello, Hannah Patricia Bennett, Jeremy Soh, Paul Kalkin, the members of my Freud Seminar, my colleagues at the Psychoanalytic Institute of Northern California, Jack Brennan, An Bulkens, Jimena Martí Haik, the administration, faculty, staff and students at the California Institute of Integral Studies: Elizabeth Markle, Emi Kojima, Judie Wexler, Elizabeth Beaven, Daniel Deslauriers, George Kich, Andrej Grubacic, and Andy Harlem; Martine Aniel, Michael Guy Thompson and the Gnosis/Esalen crew: Tonya Dowding, James Norwood, Connor Tindall, Douglas Kirsner, Rinat Tal, Andy Turkington, Scott Von, Will Hall, Nita Gage, and Fritjof Capra; Lauren Field, Nicolle Zapien, Kaisa Puhakka, Tanya Wilkinson, Amanda Morrison, Florencia Bernthal Raz, Javier Bolaños, Julieta Lucero Neirotti, German Ascani, Chris Christofferson, Chris Cerney, Matt Shields, Karl Beitel, Bernardo Isaza, Victor Bonfilio, Patrick Brooks, Andrea

Catoni, Laura Carbonara, Stephan Charbit, Carlos Disdier, Philippe Gendrault, Nicole Hsiang, and Yong Lee.

Thank you to Kate Hawes and Hannah Wright at Routledge for their expert work on this book. Their knowledge and attention to detail have been crucial to the success of this volume.

I thank my extended family here in the United States and in South America. In one way or another they have been integral parts of this endeavor. In particular, I would like to warmly acknowledge my parents, my brother, and his family. Finally, and most importantly, I would like to express my deep gratitude to the three people whose daily presence in our shared abode has helped to make life during the current pandemic not only bearable but generative.

Thomas Marchevsky: First and foremost, I express the utmost gratitude to Fernando Castrillón. It has been a great delight to work closely with him on numerous projects during the last several years. I thank Fernando for being an immensely important interlocutor. I am grateful for his ceaseless curiosity, incisive and generative words, and for the many transmissions. Our collaborations have led to a dynamic camaraderie marked by generosity and punctuated by the joke. I extend my deep appreciation to Fernando for the opportunity to co-edit this volume, for his exceptional contributions to the book and for a deep friendship shaped by the work and its improvisation.

I extend a very special thanks to Stephen Mosblech, managing editor of the *European Journal of Psychoanalysis* and key collaborator from the inception of this project. Stephen was an incredibly gracious, unfailing support. The fruition of this volume simply would not have transpired without his creativity, meticulous attention to detail, and sharpness of mind.

The big bang of this book occurred in the mind of Sergio Benvenuto, and so I express my gratitude to him for being the originary point of the text. It is a wonderful fortune to maintain a correspondence with him and I am thankful for his illuminating thoughts and contributions to the EJP.

I feel enormous gratitude for the brilliant authors included in the volume. They have articulated bold ideas at a moment when there is a lack of clear thinking about the complexities of the world, and so I thank them for making these difficult and very timely interventions.

Many thanks to Patricia Gherovici, Jamieson Webster, Todd McGowan, and Calum Neil for reviewing the text and their comments on the book.

My sincere appreciation goes to the staff at Routledge, and in particular to Kate Hawes and Hannah Wright. Our collaboration was a pleasure at all stages and the book benefited enormously from their keen insights.

I offer my innermost gratitude for the wisdom and clarity of my precious teachers Chögyal Namkhai Norbu, Yongdzin Lopön Tenzin Namdak, Tenzin Wangyal Rinpoche, Dzongsar Jamyang Khyentse Rinpoche, and Younge Khachab Rinpoche.

I extend many thanks to each of the following important individuals from various organizations including but not limited to CIIS, Saybrook, and IDC:

Philippe Gendrault, Roger Levin, Kaisa Puhakka, Alfredo Eidelzstein, Karim Dajani, Andre Patsalides Marcelo Estrada, Domenico Cosenza, Jeremy Soh, Maria Cantarini, Roberto Lazcano, Benjamin Davidson, Nathan Lupo, Paul Kalkin, Hannah Bennett, Shanna Carlson, Cecile McKenna, Steven Goodman, Andrew Harlem, Johnathan Sullivan, Danella Biondini, Elizabeth Markle, Nicolle Zapien, John Schick, Lauren Field, Stanley Krippner, Stanislav Grof, Jeanne Achterberg, Ruth Richards, Eugene Taylor, Amedeo Giorgi, Nicolle Zapien, Gabriel Rocco, Marcy Vaughn, James Munz, Kristin Aronson, Elizabeth Simpson, Fabio Andrico, Laura Evangelisti, Malcolm Smith, Martin Lowenthal, Keith Dowman, Dave Frank, Jamie Begian, Joe Diorio, George Garzone, Danilo Pérez, Shai Maestro, Christopher Morrison, Oscar Peñas, Karla Viriana, Jesse Van Fleet, Paul Nitzsche, Lungrig Gyaltsen, Nicole Turosky, and all of my students.

My heartfelt gratitude goes to Asya Grigorieva for her support throughout this project. I am thankful for the inspiration and for her radiant presence.

Finally, I wish to extend thanks to several immeasurably important connections. I cannot adequately communicate my appreciation for the generosity and influence of Isaac "El Cholo" Marchevsky, Berta Halpern, Hugo Marchevsky, Silvana Carretti, Gayle Pantaleo, Sebastian Marchevsky, Nisreen Barazi, Kamal Lahbabi, Ina Lahbabi, Bradford Harding, Margaret McMorrow, and to my extended family and friends based in Argentina and on the East Coast.

Introduction

Of pestilence, chaos, and time

Fernando Castrillón and Thomas Marchevsky
August 31, 2020

> *The past carries with it a temporal index by which it is referred to redemption.*
> (Benjamin, 1968 [1940], p. 254)

The future was not set to arrive so quickly. Yes, various global-scale calamities starting with runaway climate change were certainly waiting for us on the near horizon and had already left indelible traces of their aura in the immediacy of our daily lives. But we presumably had time; some said ten years before things became truly dreadful. So when the coronavirus[1] hit, first in China and Asia and then in Europe, rapidly spreading everywhere else in the span of a few short weeks, it seemed to take most of us by surprise: was this really happening? How could this be? Were all of the restrictions actually necessary to keep us safe? And then there is the enduring question that many of the essays in this book grapple with: was this whole imbroglio serving as a state-sanctioned excuse for an underhanded extension of its reach? Moreover, the early refrains of "when this is all over", "when we get back to normal", and "once we get on the other side of this" were ubiquitous enough that they signaled both a collective denial of the gravity of the situation and an uncertainty regarding the actual parameters of the pandemic, what possible futures might be in store for us, and how we might invest in them.

The picture, as of this writing, seems exceedingly different than just a few months ago. Not only are we still in the pandemic, but there seems no end in sight. For as much as a vaccine offers hope to so many, and while governments around the world have oriented their policies around the eventual creation and distribution of a robust, safe, and effective immunization protocol, there is also growing evidence that this hope may prove to be altogether illusory and only works to forestall other avenues for action that may in the end prove more advantageous. Going further, the ongoing pandemic has served to catalyze and *unmask* a surfeit of already active and emergent crises, most notably the seeming incapacity of most states to effectively manage the outbreaks or even to formulate any sort of coherent initial response to the developing situation. Even highly regarded approaches, such as that of Germany and New Zealand, are now being undermined by new surges of infection. Beyond its all too grim contours, the current situation leaves us with only one factor that we can all count on, namely an absolute uncertainty on all fronts: viral, economic, political, and social. Not even bleak prognoses serve as safe harbors for our anxieties. The truth of the matter is that none of us knows what is in store, such that even dire forecasts fall flat in the face of this basic uncertainty. All we can really say, in all its dim absurdity, is that there may or may not be a resolution of the viral situation and its attendant evils.

Which leaves us with no other option than to live with the pandemic and its associated ills for the (un)foreseeable future. We might come to term this state of affairs *convivirus*, perhaps a somewhat overwrought nomination, but one that speaks the name of this moment. A term, a joke or pun really, derived from the native tongue of the two editors of this volume. In Spanish, *convivir* (*convivere* in Italian) denotes living together or co-existing. From that, we are just one small step away from *convivirus*, to live together with the virus. As in to *live together*, all of us, in the face of this pestilence. But also, for us to live *with* the coronavirus, in a sort of conviviality. To embrace that the virus carries its own inhuman logic (although we cannot attribute any kind of deliberate cruelty to it) that we are forced in many ways to submit to, mitigate and orient our lives around. It is a castration that fundamentally disrupts the imagined arc of our lives, but we have not yet made it disruptive enough of hyper-modernity and digital commodity capitalism to serve as any kind of revolution (with our apologies to Žižek).

All of which gets us to the question of time, *timing* and the peculiar nature of this book. You may have noticed the date at the beginning of this introduction. You will also notice that all of the chapters include the date of original publication. Why? To answer this, consider that we are assembling this book and writing this introduction not after but in the midst of the "event". In reading and re-reading the chapters of this book, the frequent use of the phrases "for the moment" and "momentarily" becomes striking. Like the authors were either dating their writing in a way that they may not have done otherwise with other texts or in reference to other "events", or they were hedging their bets so (as) to speak, as if to say "at this moment, this is how things appear or seem to be unfolding". If anything, this would seem to signal the severe fluidity and flux of the situation, and that any pronouncements concerning this event known as the coronavirus pandemic can only be understood in their temporal context. In fact, in reviewing some of the chapters just a few months after their original date of publication in the *European Journal of Psychoanalysis*, quite a number of their observations seem hopelessly outdated, just as surely as this introduction will prove to be at some point. But this is to be expected and in fact could not have been nor cannot be any other way. Writing of the kind exhibited in this volume is necessarily problematic, full of paradox and contradiction. To write while riding or moving through the very event one is commenting on leads to all manner of strange and partially dissected formulations. In this sense, it approximates the sensibilities of a psychoanalytic session or harried dispatches from the front lines of a war, an articulating in the midst of chaos, a writing on the edge of the abyss. And for these very reasons, it is an exercise in pluck and courage. Each of these authors has staked something quite personal with their written offerings. They have chosen to speak the truth, as they understand it to be, knowing full well that they might be ridiculed or even dismissed outright for what at a later date could be read as ill-informed, judgmental, or simply short-sighted. Their daring in the face of this temporal impossibility is not something to be taken lightly. The essays in this volume, with their original dates of publication emblazoned at the beginning of each chapter, function as both chronology and testament in the face of seeming apocalypse.

In light of all this, what are we to make of this introduction? Suffice it to say that this essay, along with the rest of the book, can be read in a million different ways depending on when it is picked up by the reader. Perhaps in a more exaggerated manner than is typical, the words you are reading now can only be approached via the discomfited prism of anxieties, doubts, insights, and novel developments of the various viral moments that you are inhabiting as your eyes make their way across this page or screen. Again, it cannot be any other way.

The *European Journal of Psychoanalysis*

The following essays were all culled from two larger sets of essays focused on the coronavirus that were published in the *European Journal of Psychoanalysis* (*EJP*) starting in February 2020. The *EJP*'s long and illustrious career began 25 years ago, the brainchild of Sergio Benvenuto, a highly regarded and influential Italian psychoanalyst, philosopher, and essayist who has served as the editor in chief of the journal since its inception. Fernando Castrillón, one of the editors of this book and a longtime co-editor of the journal, has now taken up the editorial responsibilities held for so long by Benvenuto.

The *EJP* (and its previous incarnation, the *Journal of European Psychoanalysis* (*JEP*)) functions as a broad-based, fiercely independent English-language journal (with editions in Russian and Italian) dedicated to a consistently high-level engagement between Europe, the Americas, South Asia, the Middle East, and North Africa on enduring and topical questions in psychoanalysis, philosophy, the arts and contemporary social thought more broadly. The journal has published works by the leading lights of the field for 25 years and is not an organ of any one psychoanalytic school or orientation, preferring instead to provoke exchange between often alienated sub-fields and areas of inquiry. We embrace the perspective that the sensibilities engendered by psychoanalytic praxis have practical, ethical, and theoretical implications that extend far beyond clinical practice and reach into the domains of politics, activism, social policy, philosophy, cultural studies, and the social sciences. Our journal provides an international forum for the exploration of the frontiers of psychoanalytic inquiry, giving voice to diverse perspectives, research, and clinical practice which link and transform its many partial understandings.

While the journal certainly adheres to a traditional, issue-based publication format, we have also welcomed the opportunity to address more immediately pressing regional and global concerns afforded to us by the online publication of the journal via our website (www.journal-psychoanal ysis.eu/). It was through this virtual medium that the essays in this volume not only came into being but entered into an engaged and sustained conversation with each other. It is important to mention that many of these articles were originally written in French, Italian, and Spanish. We assumed the task of translating many of these texts into English so as to bring their ideas to a wider audience.

On February 26, 2020, the prominent Italian philosopher Giorgio Agamben published a short intervention in Italy titled "The Invention of an Epidemic".[2] We quickly published an English translation of the piece on our website.[3] It resulted in what can only be described as an uproar. We will attend to the details of Agamben's argument and the larger architecture of thought from which it emanated later in this introduction. What is important to note here is what his thesis and the coronavirus more generally occasioned in the pages of *EJP*. We promptly received and acquired both rapidly penned responses to Agamben's essay – and other non-Agamben-related considerations on the pestilence – by heavyweights such as Jean-Luc Nancy, Roberto Esposito, Sergio Benvenuto, Rocco Ronchi, Massimo De Carolis, Néstor Braunstein, Dany Nobus, Julia Kristeva, René Lew, Massimo Cacciari, and many other prominent intellectuals both inside and outside of Europe. We published these interventions in two "Tribunes" or sets of conversations, *Coronavirus and Philosophers* and *Psychoanalysts Facing Coronavirus*.[4]

It is difficult to describe the frenzied state of affairs that the editorial board found itself in during the roughly five-month period spanning February to June of 2020. Eschewing our traditional peer-reviewed editorial process, Sergio Benvenuto, Fernando Castrillón, and long-time editorial board member and psychoanalyst Pietro Pascarelli sorted through the various coronavirus submissions on a daily basis, choosing to only publish what we regarded as the most accomplished analyses of a rapidly developing situation.[5] As time wore on, we soon realized that these two sets of conversations had come to establish themselves as fundamentally important and highly influential forums for psychoanalytic and philosophical writing and thought on the coronavirus. This book is a selection of the very best of that uncompromising production.

Before embarking on a more detailed study of Agamben's overall philosophy, his position on the coronavirus, and the various responses to his ideas, it is useful to attend to the thought of one of the figures lurking behind many of Agamben's pronouncements and this introduction, namely, Walter Benjamin.

Benjamin's message in a bottle (and ours)

> *A chronicler who recites events without distinguishing between major and minor ones acts in accordance with the following truth: nothing that has ever happened should be regarded as lost for history. To be sure, only a redeemed mankind receives the fullness of its past – which is to*

say, only for a redeemed mankind has its past become citable in all its moments. Each moment it has lived becomes a citation á l'ordre du jour *– and that day is Judgement Day.*

(Benjamin, 1968 [1940], p. 254)

It is worthwhile to consider what it is of the past, both immediate and remote, that the authors and editors of this book are so furtively attempting to cite and keep alive, and towards what end? Benjamin's magisterial essay, "Theses on the Philosophy of History", is revelatory in this respect. Hewing closely, both knowingly and unwittingly, to the various positions he outlines in that celebrated text, the various chronologies of this volume, and the historical articulation of the past embedded in this particular essay do not aim to give accounts of the pandemic and the circumstances surrounding the emergence of the essays in the manner of "what actually and factually happened". We leave others to find succor in that bordello. Instead we opt to "seize hold of memory as it flashes up at a moment of danger", in our case an extended, rupturing moment of peril encased in an immediate, heterogeneous now that we blast out of the "continuum of history" (Benjamin, 1968 [1940], pp. 255–261). Individually and as a group, these essays serve as a message in a bottle to both ourselves and the future. A collective scream signaling again and again that any forgetting of this particular moment in the service of "progress" or "resolution" can only function to lead us more quickly to our final grave. In their best instances, these chapters establish a constellated and fraught linking with subterranean histories that have been banished to the margins by the "victors" and their history-tellers. In this way, they work against a reactionary and stupid conformism that threatens to eclipse previous moments of struggle, thereby redeeming an evaporated past so as to make it available, citable, and even alive.

Our fervent wish is that this book serve, by virtue of its uncompromising focus on this moment of crisis, as a mechanism for later generations to tear asunder the continuum of history and perhaps to redeem the failed efforts of our plague-stricken time and even their own. The movement is twofold, a progression into the past that undergirds a reaching into a future unknown and in doubt.

Going further, could we argue that this pandemic-induced enormous pause to life (as we have known it) may very well come to break open the closed, fateful, and guilt-laden box of the historicist's homogeneous empty-time, allowing us a Messianic moment of disruption, rupture, discontinuity à la Benjamin? The official, linear histories of the pandemic are already being written, narratives are already being sanctimoniously stitched together (pre-pandemic/pandemic/post-pandemic) that kill off the dead yet again, carving out ready-made mass graves, final abodes of the anonymous and the unseen, thereby cheating the future and ourselves of their once vital trace. But it does not have to be so. The supreme catastrophe is *not* that we fail to make it out of the pandemic and resume our previous lives, but that we in fact do so in such a way that we leave the pandemic "behind" us and squander yet another grand opportunity to change the course of things. Hell is not so much what is happening now, as calamitous as things have become. Disaster's feast had been properly arranged long before Wuhan. If there is such a thing that we can call Hope, it *may* come to arise from the unruly ashes of our current experience and not from an orderly return to what we had before.

Giorgio Agamben and the state of (his) exception

> *The tradition of the oppressed teaches us that the "state of emergency" in which we live is not the exception but the rule. We must attain to a conception of history that is in keeping with this insight.*

(Benjamin, 1968 [1940], p. 257)

Any reader of Agamben's work will quickly realize that the architecture of his thought is highly predicated on a very particular reading of Benjamin, Martin Heidegger, and Michel Foucault. While this is important to bear in mind, the aim of this introduction does not necessitate an exhaustive rendition of Agamben's work nor an examination of how he reconfigures the thought of the above three philosophers into novel forms of theoretical expression. Instead, our efforts will focus on tracing the more salient aspects of his thought and their import for the various essays of this volume that engage with his assertions on the coronavirus.

It is worthwhile to note that the early days of the pandemic brought with them the notion that governmental responses to the pestilence and Agamben's pronouncements regarding them, provided a near-perfect opportunity to put his ideas regarding the state of exception, biopolitics, bare or naked life, and *homo sacer* more generally, on the stand. This *experimentum crucis* took place in various venues, including the *EJP*.

However, there is more to this scene, for it is also the case that the pandemic, the response by governments, and the in-vivo examination of Agamben's thought find their grounding in a collective reckoning with the horrors of World War II and the ensuing sequalae. As Benjamin Bennett outlines in his foreword to Laurence A. Rickels's three-volume tome, *Nazi Psychoanalysis*, "Nazism cannot be isolated in the structure of modernity, that no element of modernity can be thought adequately without thinking its Nazi component" (2002, p. xii). Which is to say that Nazism, and the absolute terrors it brought to bear or revealed more fully, reside in every nook and cranny of modernity, such that a consideration of Agamben's pronouncements regarding state responses to the pandemic necessarily involves a reexamination of these reviled and abject features of our not-too-distant past.

By way of beginning our engagement with Agamben's thought, we will work with a short intervention of his from May 11, 2020, titled "Biosecurity and Politics" (originally published in Italian[6] and translated into English[7]). This article is useful in that it succinctly states so much of what Agamben noted elsewhere during the course of the pandemic, thereby allowing us to engage his work and to bring forward comments that are echoed throughout this volume. We can then use these as a springboard for a more detailed examination of some of his major concepts, such as biopolitics, state of exception, naked (or bare) life, and *homo sacer*. For example, he notes:

> If already in the gradual decline of political ideologies and beliefs, the reasons for security had allowed citizens to accept the limitations of freedoms that they were not previously willing to accept, biosecurity has been shown to be capable of presenting the absolute cessation of all political activity and social relations as the maximum form of civic participation. We have thus witnessed the paradox of left-wing organizations, traditionally accustomed to claiming rights and denouncing violations of the constitution, accepting without reservation the limitations of freedom decided by ministerial decrees deprived of any legality and which even fascism had never dreamed of being able to impose.
>
> (Agamben, 2020c)

We will only be reiterating a sentiment found throughout several, though certainly not all, of the following essays when we say that Agamben's mistake here is in confusing his conception of biopolitics (more on this below) and the material facts of an all too real virus. Yes, certain states may very well be using the pandemic to advance novel forms of repressive governance, but that observation does not negate the actuality of the coronavirus itself. Put another way, denying the infectious logic of the virus does not serve to advance his claims regarding biopolitics or the nature of contemporary states.

Agamben's confusion on this point joins with another feature of his thought, namely, the universalizing nature of his theorizing which ends up transforming many of his pronouncements into blanket statements devoid of specificity and nuance. For example, in the same essay, he notes:

> What Zylberman described in 2013 has now been verified accurately. It is obvious that, beyond the emergency situation linked to a certain virus, which in the future may give way to another, what is in question is the design of a paradigm of government whose effectiveness far exceeds that of all forms of government that the political history of the West had hitherto known.
>
> (Agamben, 2020c)

Putting aside the possibility that the ascendency of this novel paradigm of government may indeed be taking place in some areas of the globe, it is certainly not the case in places like the United States, Brazil, and the Philippines, whose respective governments are abdicating the throne of the *bios* (more on this further down) and are instead falling back on an unmasked *display* of their repressive capacities. In other words, and to use the United States as the premier example of this, instead of *utilizing* the pandemic and concerns regarding biosecurity to extend its reach and introduce restrictive political measures that were unthinkable just a few months ago, the federal government has relinquished this opportunity so as to exert its power via an already overwhelming repressive apparatus – a long-standing feature of North American statecraft, as exemplified by the recent and blatant use of heavily armed federal Department of Homeland Security agents to violently crush mostly peaceful protests against the relentless police killings of African Americans.

While Agamben's totalizing generalizations and misapprehension on critical points can often dilute the overall power of his critique, it is also true that we cannot so easily dismiss the entirety of his approach, especially if we change some of its temporal dimensions. Case in point, Agamben ends this same essay with the following words:

> After politics has been replaced by the economy, even now it, in order to govern, will have to be integrated into the new paradigm of biosecurity, to which all other requirements will have to be sacrificed. It is legitimate to ask whether such a society can still define itself as human, or whether the loss of sensitive relationships, face, friendship, love, can be truly compensated by an abstract and presumed fictitious health security.
>
> (Agamben, 2020c)

Surely it can be argued that many of us reflect on this set of losses and experience the pain that they bring. It is undeniably hurtful, but the opposite, as in proceeding as "normal",[8] is far worse. It is full-on death. We must certainly, and without flinching, name the losses we have incurred, mourn them, and work to, at some specified point, re-inhabit those spaces forbidden to us by the infectious logic of the virus. It is vital that we not lose sight of these points of injury, for they work as our base of resistance and in service of the urgent task of reclaiming these forsaken spaces and functions once the calculus of infection, freedom of movement, and exchange has undergone a transformation. What we can take from Agamben, among other things, is a commitment to dispel any fiction of biosecurity as a support for new forms of governance that might have come to roost on our collective shores during this period of the pandemic. It will be decisive to do exactly this, and in that way, it may very well turn out to be an Agambenian moment.

Bearing all this in mind, let us now turn to a more detailed exploration of four of Agamben's concepts that form the contested terrain of engagement for many of the essays that follow.

*Biopolitics/state of exception/naked (or bare) life/*homo sacer[9]

Agamben's ontological theory of sovereignty and his theory of the state serve as our points of departure. Working against some aspects of contemporary thought, he makes a direct link between ontology, the problem of sovereignty, and the state, which is also a way of saying that the latter's existence does not necessarily depend on particular components of state discourse or even the law. For Agamben, sovereignty is the *sine qua non* of social life. Taking this idea further, we see that there is an immediate relationship between state sovereignty and life, such that the state's manner of conceiving has direct implications for how life is understood, managed, and catalogued.

Sovereignty expresses itself and establishes its power via its abilities of exception and exclusion, which give rise to the juridical order. By virtue of this capacity to decide who is allowed entry to the body politic – and just as importantly, who is kept out – sovereignty lends itself to the development of the state. State power, then, is premised on making humans vulnerable and abject. Agamben does not regard the state as beneficent but as a totalizing power with absolute say over life and death. To be part of the body politic, one must submit totally and be made vulnerable.

In Agamben's telling, sovereignty relates to life in two different ways, the *bios* (the form or manner in which life is lived) and *zoē* (the biological fact of life). The latter term is often referred to as *bare* or *naked life*[10] and includes the animality of human existence. In his view, what has come to predominate our contemporary experience is the state's relation to life as naked life. In other words, the state sees life at its most basic as naked, and reserves for itself the capacity to transform it into *bios* or life invested with political recognition and representation, or at the very least to nullify the distinction between the two. In other words, state sovereignty decides who is recognized as "human" with an ethically significant life, and who is catalogued as having nothing other than naked life and thereby devoid of the kind of "rights" and protections afforded to full citizens.[11] Moreover, a state's declaration of "exception" allows it to strip away anyone's political recognition and representation.

The figure of *homo sacer* (sacred/taboo/execrated human) is the distilled locus of naked life. Outside the realm of the law and valued life, this figure is vulnerable to being killed with impunity but cannot be sacrificed. Interestingly, the sovereign and the *homo sacer* function as two ends of a concave mirror, existing both within and outside the law. What is important for us to recognize here, per Agamben, is that life under state control necessarily means an ever-present danger of being declared *homo sacer*. Despite all the assurances of modern liberalism, this capacity of modern states to declare anyone *homo sacer* is not only a fundament of actual state practice but is increasingly coming to play a crucial role via *states of exception*, which allow whole populations and segments of the larger society to be reduced to naked life (e.g. migrant camps in the United States and Europe, Abu Ghraib, and Guantanamo Bay). What is critical to underline here is that the state's capacity to institute a state of exception that suspends normal legal guarantees, protections and basic rights can be applied to anyone or any group at any time, thereby implying that everyone is vulnerable or at risk. Moreover, these states of exception to the usual rule of law can be applied to an entire society, which is the concern that Agamben raises in relation to the restrictions imposed by various states in response to the coronavirus.

For Agamben, sovereignty as such eventually leads to Auschwitz, where the state of exception is made permanent in both time and space. In this way, the Nazi death camps signal our collective future, since it is there that the ontological nature of sovereignty reveals its ultimate endpoint. As subjects of contemporary states and the unfolding of the logic of sovereignty, we are always moving towards Auschwitz. Indeed, for him, whatever distinction may have held between the camp and the larger social field has collapsed. The only possible alternative is a full-scale assault on sovereignty itself.

It is this particular aspect of Agamben's theorizing that leads him and others who share this line of thought to take often unpopular and derided positions. His pronouncements on the coronavirus, examined above and throughout many of the following essays, are just one example of this tendency. For him, the horrors of the Holocaust are always waiting to emerge yet again and are not marginal or remote aspects of contemporary life but very possible and central features of how contemporary states and sovereignty function. Stated differently, governmental restrictions on human movement and exchange in response to the coronavirus are understood as ontological in nature rather than contingent phenomena with no underlying logic or veiled dynamic at play, and demonstrate an increasing propensity for the (state of) exception to become the rule.

In terms of *biopolitics*, it was Foucault who recognized a shift in modernity whereby the state increasingly came to assume the task of supervising and regulating biological, human life itself. The inauguration, beginning in the 17th century, of what he terms *biopower*, a regularizing technology of power that apportions human life according to value and utility, signals the rise of biopolitics.

While Foucault maintains a distinction between sovereign power and disciplinary biopower, with the latter supplanting the former in his account, Agamben argues that sovereign power is always already biopolitical, since it is naked life that functions as the point of convergence for political order in modernity. Hence, for Agamben, biopower is nothing other than a continuation of sovereign power, as evidenced by an increased reliance by governments around the world on the state of exception and the rise of naked life as a terminal point for increasingly greater segments of human society.

Book layout: a reader's guide

Organization and general lines of argumentation

The book is segmented in three parts: Part I (Philosophers speak), Part II (Philosophers act) and Part III (Psychoanalysts speak). The following is a brief outline of the organization of the text and the main contours of its arguments.

Part I is structured around a series of conversations regarding Giorgio Agamben's controversial analysis of the coronavirus pandemic. Given legal constraints regarding publishing rights, Agamben's complete texts were not included in this book.

The necessary context for Agamben's pronouncements regarding the pandemic is provided above in the first part of the introduction. The reader is also invited to read Agamben's coronavirus related articles by using the web links provided in the references section at the end of this introductory chapter.

The opening chapter of the book sets the stage with an excerpt from Foucault's *Discipline and Punish* and is followed by several discussions by eminent contemporary philosophers. Their arguments pivot around three main problems: (1) articulating definitional issues regarding Agamben's key terms including *biopolitics*, *bare* or *naked life*, and *states of exception*; (2) addressing the extent to which Agamben succeeds or fails to provide a coherent account of the pandemic; and (3) clarifying points of disagreement about Agamben's conclusions in order to develop more rigorous analyses of the various social and political crises at hand. Within this fruitful set of "conversations" we find divergent points of view. Some philosophers discount Agamben's perspective altogether, while others point out its partial veracity recognizing the necessity of extending the discussion in order to more adequately conceptualize the complex conditions of the present crisis.

Part II comprises a collection of texts from distinguished philosophers bringing forth perspectives from different parts of the globe ranging from Europe to the Indian subcontinent. The authors continue to elaborate key themes from Part I and also broaden the discourse to a variety of other philosophical issues. These writings are at times very personal accounts of the conditions on the ground as it were, and at other times they provide coordinates by which to think about the most severe political and societal consequences of this pandemic: dread and anxiety, the fear of contagion, the dissolution of symbolic ties, the effects of social isolation, the toll of innumerable deaths and amassment of bodies, and the interruption of interment rites.

Part III is a collection of writings by distinguished psychoanalysts who articulate frontier positions in the field. Analytic writing as a form has been crucial since the inception of psychoanalysis, but its import is perhaps more readily graspable now than ever before. In this period of global crisis and major flux, the textual tradition allows analysts to inscribe symbolic commitments and to establish new positions via the word. In contradistinction to the discourses of the master and the university, psychoanalytic writing functions in service of the discourse of the analyst, as formulated by Jacques Lacan. As such, the analyst accepts a particular position vis-à-vis the lack, thereby allowing the elaboration of the speaking subject of the unconscious. Necessarily incomplete and full of holes, the writings in this section avoid the trappings of totalizing discourses. In a period of incalculable chaos, it is natural to wish to take solace in knowledge, but this is no time to give way to fantasies of certainty. There will be no such victories because there is no one viral enemy and no one war; there is no cure because there is no one disease. What we have is a convergence of pandemics: political, economic, social, and last but not least, the coronavirus. The authors in this section speak to the necessity of inventiveness in psychoanalysis. This creativity is what can allow for new conceptualizations of the analytic work that can thereby speak to the rapidly shifting circumstances of our time. The authors represent a psychoanalytic sensibility that is characterized by the desire to continue listening and finding ways to hear progressively more. These analysts are *being with* Covid, or to put it another way, they are *co-void* . . . desiring as they stare into the abyss.

Chapter introductions

Part I: philosophers speak

The book commences with an excerpt from Michel Foucault's *Discipline and Punish: The Birth of the Prison*. This chapter introduces many themes developed throughout the book providing a backdrop of key philosophical issues. This account of one of the "great plagues" of the 17th century provides a strikingly relevant description of the ways in which power and social control both become determined by and determine the consequences of pandemics. Foucault's haunting description of quarantine and surveillance opens us to enduring questions of how the plague can set in motion mechanisms of power and the structuration of a disciplined society.

Chapter 2, "A Viral Exception", begins a philosophical exchange revolving around the work of Giorgio Agamben. In this chapter, French philosopher Jean-Luc Nancy takes a critical position against Agamben's early pronouncements regarding the coronavirus (see above for a summary of Agamben's stance). Nancy argues that the current crisis cannot be understood simply as another pretext for a "state of exception". With this warning regarding Agamben's reductive reading of the pandemic, Nancy invites us to think beyond claims of governmental misuse of power. In what he calls "viral exception", Nancy extends the notion of exception to the domains of biology, technoscience, and culture.

In Chapter 3, "Cured to the Bitter End", Italian philosopher Roberto Esposito formulates a critical response to Nancy, stressing that a link between biological life and politics, or biopolitics, is at the essence of conflicts in contemporary social life. Esposito charges Nancy with refusing biopolitics and thereby failing to grasp why these terms must function inseparably. The chapter concludes with the notion that current political disorder is not an attempt by leaders to seize control and power (i.e. a convenient pretext for declaring "a state of exception") but instead should be interpreted as symptomatic of the ineptitude of a failed state.

Chapter 4, "Riposte to Roberto Esposito", is Jean-Luc Nancy's succinct rejoinder about his rejection of the term "biopolitics". In a swift deconstruction, Nancy indicates that the terms "biology" and "politics" are on their own ill-defined and so concludes that their amalgamation is pointless.

In Chapter 5, philosophers Divya Dwivedi and Shaj Mohan explore a deepening crisis regarding the value of human life. "The Community of the Forsaken: A Response to Agamben and Nancy" further contextualizes the philosophical questions addressed in the previous chapters by introducing issues of temporality and various paradigms of exception. The authors articulate the ethical implications of the movement from god or "theo-technologies" to our present era of "techno-theology" wherein "we are entrusting the machine with the determination of ends". Moreover, Dwivedi and Mohan explore the latent conditions that make possible the emergence of a "state of exception" during this particular historical moment. At a time during which biopolitics unfold with machinic momentum, the authors raise incisive questions concerning being, death, and responsibility.

Chapter 6, written by Italian philosopher Rocco Ronchi, opens with a keen insight: that the unknowns of the pandemic should not be conflated with what is fervently denied, namely our finitude (in point of fact, death is the only thing about which we can be certain). It is problematic to reduce our concerns about the virus to how likely we are to die from it, though the risks loom and should not be suppressed. Falling for this trap of fear would be to negate the actual antagonisms of *this singular event*. The pandemic may have merit, as the title "The Virtues of the Virus" suggests, but if truth is to be discovered amidst its chaos, it will be possible only to the extent that we examine the unique factors leading to and that are generated by the circumstances. This logic is legible right on the surface – the spread of the virus reveals incompetence, corruption, and exploitation. Ronchi argues that all of this points directly to the fact that politics must be brought to a place of primacy and such that it can assume its rightful functions. He also reminds us that this is an occasion by which to recognize our limits and that we cannot rule over the natural world. Ronchi argues that if we are to traverse this calamity, the virtuous path will be that of harnessing our political powers so as to live in recognition of our interdependence, thereby forging a way toward freedom.

In Chapter 7, "The Threat of Contagion", Italian philosopher Massimo De Carolis articulates the question of the hour, one intensified by each moment of prolonged isolation measures: what kinds of new social arrangements will we be forced to negotiate (and for how long)? Will there be a perpetual tension between biological survival and new risks in sociality? In sum, what price will we need to pay for the preservation of the social bond? De Carolis aptly points out that the deterioration of the symbolic order is not a new problem, and that its decline has many antecedents predating the coronavirus. Thus, the author asserts that what is important to consider regarding sociality today and compounded with already existing complications, is that we face a novel set of issues consequent to the conditions of the current crisis.

In Chapter 8, "What Carries Us On", Shaj Mohan explores the decline of metaphysics and the contradictions of hypophysics, and points out how these each lead to impasses. Tracing the work of Kant, Nietzsche, Heidegger, Gandhi, Nancy, and others, Mohan addresses how we have reached a point of "inability to distinguish between good and evil". Given the vexed problems of morality and the deleterious conditions of the pandemic as a backdrop, the question of "what carries us on" takes on a radical significance. Mohan extends a response to the problem of what makes life worth living: the shared experience of solitude and *mysterium tremendum*.

In Chapter 9, "The Obscure Experience", Shaj Mohan extends his argument from the previous chapter by noting: "we assume from the common uses of the terms 'natural' and 'normal' that nature is a set of norms". In this set of reflections, Mohan invites us to reconsider the assumptions and terms that form the basis for biopolitics and "global circulatory systems". Along these lines, he argues that the notion of an "idyllic a priori" subverts our freedom. Mohan concludes by indicating the importance of "co-belonging" as a necessary step to the democratization of the world.

Chapter 10, "Agamben, the Virus, and the Biopolitical: A Riposte", written by cultural studies professor Zsuzsa Baross, takes a sharply critical stance against Agamben's assessment of the pandemic by dismantling various terms including "biopolitics" and by indicating that current forces at work cannot be simply reduced to the notion of a "state of exception". She argues that what characterizes the political responses to the pandemic is best understood as "an extreme (exceptional) self-defensive measure and immune reaction". Furthermore, the problem of "bare life" is dialectized in relation to Deleuze's concept of "*a* life". In the context of the dire medical crisis of this pandemic, Baross illustrates the practically seamless movement from the treatment of "*a* life" in its singularity to its sudden expendability.

Chapter 11, written by Jean-Luc Nancy, articulates the coordinates by which Europe has positioned itself with regard to the pandemic, highlighting a contrast between how it and other regions of the world have handled the crisis. In "A Much Too Human Virus", Nancy explores the consequences of globalism, and the limits and dangers of political and technical dominance. The central question concerns the appearance and status of the phenomena of the coronavirus in that what seem to be intrusions from the outside might in reality be more aptly understood as human products (*outrusions?*). Ultimately, this chapter confronts us with the disconcerting notion that our role in the production of and response to the pandemic may be evidence of what is inexorably human and therefore insurmountable.

Chapter 12, "The Return of Antigone: Burial Rites in Pandemic Times" is an unflinching look at disruptions to inhumation and its effects on society. Using the allegory of Sophocles's *Antigone*, Argentine/Mexican psychoanalyst Néstor Braunstein raises fundamental issues regarding shifting interment practices and offers keen observations with respect to the treatment of the dead during the pandemic. The crux of Braunstein's arguments concern the cultural importance of burial rites. Contemplating these rituals, he writes: "they make death a social event and not an individual avatar". Thus, in the absence of burial rites we are forced to confront that we must not only live with the death of the body, but also a second death or "two deaths". Beyond the passing of a life, there is an-Other loss consequent to the prohibition of burial rites, and this interdiction of the symbolic restructures society.

Part II: philosophers act

In Chapter 13, "One Health and One Home: On the Biopolitics of Covid-19", Miguel Vatter, professor of political science, elucidates two salient issues concerning the pandemic. One is the necessity of rethinking viral trajectories crossing over species and what this implies for social stratifications. A second key theme is that of lockdown measures taken and what means will be advanced to achieve political ends. Vatter invites us to rethink the relation between our homes, health, and humanity, and warns of the perils of resurrecting the state as savior in times of vulnerability. Against the mistake of seeking false assurances, Vatter marks another option: submission to nature's law as a path to Humanity.

In Chapter 14, "The Italian Laboratory: Rethinking Debt in Viral Times", Italian philosopher Elettra Stimilli tells us "we need new words". Pointing out the lacunae in Agamben's theory and the economics of Italian debt, she argues that our conception of the coronavirus must extend beyond merely treating it as a biological phenomenon. To this end, she argues for the necessity of accountability for the roles played by global capitalism and ecological catastrophes. Amidst financial crises and the invocation of war rhetoric to combat the virus, Stimilli signals that these conditions call for political innovation.

In Chapter 15, "*Vitam Instituere*", written by Roberto Esposito, explores the impact of the pandemic on social relations. More than just a threat to "bare life", the pandemic encroaches on the interactional structures that generate meaning and significance for each of us individually and in relation to each other. Bearing in mind the breakdown of social conventions, Esposito invites us to examine shifting notions of proxemics and sociality. Paradoxically, a reorientation to space through practices of isolation may be precisely what reveals new forms of solidarity.

In Chapter 16, "Communovirus", Jean-Luc Nancy makes an argument for the potential generated by the coronavirus crisis. Like Esposito in the previous chapter, he communicates that being in isolation is in fact a way of *being with*. The pandemic brings us together in unexpected ways and in this sense is a great equalizer. It "communizes" insofar as it makes increasingly explicit the actuality of our interdependence. Nancy argues that what is at stake is nothing less than the potential for our liberation. In this moment of crisis, he suggests that there exists the possibility of a disarticulation of capitalist values and therefore the possibility of a movement from the accumulation of capital to the transcendence of the individual.

In Chapter 17, "Satanization of Man. The Pandemic and the Wound of Narcissism", Italian psychoanalyst and philosopher Sergio Benvenuto speaks incisively about the dangers of ideology and its effects during this pandemic. This chapter covers much ground, starting with our refusal of death and ending with the limits of science and objectivity. Benvenuto tells us, "the death of god leaves *the place* of divinity vacant", through which humans narcissistically attempt to recoup a loss of omnipotence by taking the place of god. The notion of Man as god introduces its logical counterpart, namely, the "Satanization of

Man". The text examines the dangers of these imaginary positions and the consequences of Man's inability to accept limits to enjoyment.

Chapter 18, "A Viral Revaluation of All Values?" is British psychoanalyst Dany Nobus's at once personal and critical reflection on the gravity of the pandemic. Naming the social, economic, and political contradictions exposed by the situation, he turns toward the antecedents and underpinnings of the coronavirus crisis. In a chilling conclusion, Nobus alerts us to the very real possibility that the horrors of the pandemic may not suffice to produce a reappraisal of our priorities. This chapter elucidates a disconcerting paradox; namely, that if the pandemic is at some point contained but without the supplementary work of an authentic revaluation process, even greater catastrophes may transpire.

In Chapter 19, French psychoanalyst Julia Kristeva is interviewed about the pandemic and articulates the importance of a "revaluation of life", thus forming a textual link to Nobus's chapter. "Humanity Is Rediscovering Existential Solitude, the Meaning of Limits, and Mortality" examines the coronavirus and three other plagues of hypermodernity: (1) insufferable loneliness, (2) boundless narcissism, and (3) the denial of death. With spontaneity and clarity, Kristeva puts words to pervasive forms of angst and questions our relation to pleasure and sexuality, thereby pointing the way to a rethinking of our ethics.

Chapter 20, "A Flight Indestinate", by Divya Dwivedi, is a meditation on the concepts of time and speed and an invitation to reflect on what is needed in times of pandemics. On these issues, Dwivedi provides an evocative image: "The pandemic has occasioned certain exchanges of speeds such that this world machine is seizing up like an overheated engine. What care does this moment need?" Dwivedi's answer is developed by her notion of "indestinacy", a neologism that evokes as of yet unthought possibilities and how these potentialities may shape our destiny.

Part III: psychoanalysts speak

Chapter 21, "Psychoanalysis, Too, Will Never Be the Same", intervenes on the terrain of the analytic clinic. In this thought-provoking chapter, Néstor Braunstein creates an aperture for exploring current transformations in the field of psychoanalysis and subjectivity. Further, he delimits the function of psychoanalysis. Braunstein tells us that psychoanalysis as a praxis addresses the particulars of the subject and in transference to the analyst; this a timely reminder given the temptation to extend psychoanalysis beyond its scope, particularly at a moment replete with unanswered questions. Further, Braunstein theorizes the virus as a new type of *object a* and reflects on the consequences for the analytic session occasioned by the deployment of new technologies in clinical work.

In Chapter 22, "Politics of the Letter. Screened Speech is the Foreclosure of the Littoral of the Letter", French psychoanalyst René Lew explores the causes and consequences of disruptions to the social link consequent to pandemic related distancing and isolation measures. In reference to the previous chapter by Braunstein, the author further investigates these issues in an examination of contemporary technical adaptations being made in the psychoanalytic clinic. Lew argues that use of the screen or phone diminishes the ambiguity of speech, and that the "real void" replaces the "symbolic void" wherein a transformed *object a* loses the lack.

In Chapter 23, "*Hestiation*. Our Life After Coronavirus", Sergio Benvenuto reflects on a wide range of cultural shifts, including changes in sociality and the transformation of the home into the site of the workplace. Benvenuto notes that the temporality of these changes (and the possibility of their permanence) is uncertain and insists on the importance of adaptability. Change and innovation is difficult to accept, he tells us, given our tendency to privilege familiar modes of being and doing things. As Benvenuto ably points out, the question is not that of when things return to normal but rather of undoing presuppositions that preclude new ways of thinking, working, and being in a world that has been indelibly altered by the pandemic.

In Chapter 24, "The Virus and the Unconscious. Diary From the Quarantine", Sergio Benvenuto makes astute observations about the impact of fallacious beliefs on everyday life during the pandemic. With humor and wit, Benvenuto reviews a series of recent phenomena: the faulty assumption that withstanding adversity necessarily generates strength, the frenzied fixation on toilet paper, the confusion about what populations are most vulnerable, and the propaganda about vectors of transmission. As a countermeasure to widely held misconceptions about the virus, Benvenuto offers two powerful antidotes: a turn to statistical analyses for an objective view of the realities of the virus and the examination of unconscious mechanisms sustaining irrational beliefs.

Chapter 25, "Talking Cure by Phone During the Lockdown", authored by French psychoanalyst Monique Lauret, dives into the polemics of conducting analytic work outside of the consulting room, noting the dogmatism of those who maintain that such practices are in fact not psychoanalysis. This compelling chapter takes up several of the same key themes as the contribution by Lew, among them the issue of what may be lost in the transmission of speech via the medium of the phone. To this point, Lauret states: "the message, whether true or ambiguous, aims at . . . the presence of the other as an absolute Other." With this assertion, she indicates that the deciphering of messages to the Other by phone remains a possibility, implying that the onus of doing so is on the analyst. Further, Lauret offers a window into her own clinic work; despite the pandemic (or perhaps because of it), analysands come to speak intimately about anxiety, life, and death.

In the final chapter of the book, "The Truth About Coronavirus", Canadian psychoanalyst and professor of sociology Duane Rousselle provides a provocative account of the place of psychoanalysis during this crisis. The "talking cure", properly speaking, is no cure at all for a nightmarish pandemic. Far from a panacea, psychoanalysis makes possible "access to a truth which determines us and might be put to social use", explains Rousselle. The closing chapter makes direct reference to Foucault (with whom the book begins) and

Agamben (catalyst for many of the conversations in the book) – Rousselle dissents on reading the mechanisms and functioning of capitalism strictly according to Agamben's terms. The problem for Rousselle is that concepts such as "bare life" and "state of exception" remain decontextualized, or more precisely, that they are deployed "without situating these techniques as responses to the new paradigms of jouissance". As the book's final cut, this chapter has a retroactive effect. Rousselle punctuates an end point, and with this we can make further use of the previous chapters so as continue the arduous, uncertain, but nevertheless essential work of elaborating positions in an era of confusion and disorder.

(In)conclusion

Properly speaking, there can be no conclusion to either this essay or the implications of the pandemic that currently rages in our midst. This moment of viral outbreak, by which we mean both the coronavirus and the various essays of this book, vigorously resist the facile way in which most edited volumes of this sort reach a moment of closure. There is no resolution here.

In a similar manner to the chapters that follow, this introduction is a snapshot of a moment all too replete with complexity and dread. It captures certain lines of flight, only to forsake others of equal or even greater importance. We miss the mark the moment we strike words on the page. This is always the dilemma posed by the task of writing; incompleteness haunts the entire body of this text. And it is in this spirit of solidarity afforded by an all too obvious lack that we offer this book to you, dear reader. Our grand hope is that your desire may come to fill the countless crevices and cracks that hold it all together.

Notes

1   While the official name for the virus is SARS-CoV-2, and Covid-19 for the disease, we are staying with the more popular, albeit inaccurate rendition of both the virus and the disease as the coronavirus. As well, most of the authors in this collection also refer to this confluence of virus and disease as the coronavirus.
2   Agamben (2020a). www.quodlibet.it/giorgio-agamben-l-invenzione-di-un-epidemia
3   www.journal-psychoanalysis.eu/coronavirus-and-philosophers/
4   All the original essays that we collected for this book have been removed from the *EJP* website, in accordance with an agreement with Routledge. However, all the other "Tribune" essays that we did not include in this book are still available on the website, including the initial Agamben translation that we refer to above.
5   We, of course, retained our peer-review procedure for all other, non-coronavirus submissions to the journal.
6   Agamben (2020c). www.quodlibet.it/giorgio-agamben-biosicurezza
7   https://medium.com/@ddean3000/biosecurity-and-politics-giorgio-agamben-396f9ab3b6f4
8   It is crucial to note that Agamben's words on the matter can easily be read as an advocation for continuing as before. For example, in his initial essay (dated February 26, 2020) that we referred to above, he deems the pandemic restrictions as "frenetic, irrational and

entirely unfounded emergency measures adopted against an alleged epidemic of corona-virus" (www.journal-psychoanalysis.eu/coronavirus-and-philosophers/).

9 The following rendition of Agamben's ideas is gleaned from the following texts: *Homo Sacer: Sovereign Power and Bare Life* (1998); *Remnants of Auschwitz: The Witness and the Archive. Homo Sacer III* (1999); *Means Without End: Notes on Politics* (2000); and *State of Exception* (2005). Our analysis of Foucault relies on his following two texts: *The History of Sexuality, Volume 1: An Introduction* (1990) and *"Society Must Be Defended", Lectures at the Collège de France, 1975–76* (2003).

10 The term used by Agamben in Italian is *nuda vita*, most directly translated into English as *naked life*, which is also the preferred term used by Cesare Casarino, an early translator of Agamben's work into English ("Form of Life" in *Radical Thought in Italy: A Potential Politics* [1996]). We find that *naked life* is a more faithful English-language rendition of the stark tenor of the original term in Italian. Although it bears mentioning that Agamben's *nuda vita* is itself a translation (of sorts) of Benjamin's *das bloße Leben*, which in several respects does not coincide with Agamben's rendering into Italian. For more on this thorny topic, see Carlo Salzani's "From Benjamin's *bloßes Leben* to Agamben's *Nuda Vita*: A Genealogy" in *Towards the Critique of Violence: Walter Benjamin and Giorgio Agamben* (2015).

11 It should be noted, however, that in Agamben's view the distinction between naked life and politically recognized life is dissolving as the logic of state sovereignty unfolds over time.

References

Agamben, G. (1996). Form of life. In P. Virno & M. Hardt (Eds.), *Radical thought in Italy: A potential politics* (pp. 151–155). University of Minnesota Press.

Agamben, G. (1998). *Homo sacer: Sovereign power and bare life*. Stanford University Press.

Agamben, G. (1999). *Remnants of Auschwitz: The witness and the archive. Homo sacer III*. Zone Books.

Agamben, G. (2000). *Means without end: Notes on politics*. University of Minnesota Press.

Agamben, G. (2005). *State of exception*. University of Chicago Press.

Agamben, G. (2020a, February 26). L'invenzione di un'epidemia. *Quodlibet*. www.quodlibet.it/giorgio-agamben-l-invenzione-di-un-epidemia

Agamben, G. (2020b, February 26). The invention of an epidemic. *The European Journal of Psychoanalysis*. www.journal-psychoanalysis.eu/coronavirus-and-philosophers/

Agamben, G. (2020c, May 11). Biosicurezza e politica. *Quodlibet*. www.quodlibet.it/giorgio-agamben-biosicurezza

Agamben, G. (2020d, May 11). Biosecurity and politics. *Medium*. https://medium.com/@ddean3000/biosecurity-and-politics-giorgio-agamben-396f9ab3b6f4

Benjamin, W. (1968). Theses on the philosophy of history. In H. Arendt (Ed.), *Illuminations: Essays & reflections* (pp. 253–264). Schocken Books. (Original work published 1940)

Bennett, B. (2002). Foreword. In L. A. Rickels (Ed.), *Nazi psychoanalysis, volume I: Only psychoanalysis won the war* (pp. VII–XIII). University of Minnesota Press.

Foucault, M. (1990). *The history of sexuality, volume 1: An introduction*. Vintage Books.

Foucault, M. (2003). *"Society must be defended", lectures at the Collège de France, 1975–76*. Picador.

Salzani, C. (2015). From Benjamin's "bloßes Leben" to Agamben's "Nuda Vita": A genealogy. In B. Moran & C. Salzani (Eds.), *Towards the critique of violence: Walter Benjamin and Giorgio Agamben* (pp. 109–123). Bloomsbury Academic.

Part I
Philosophers speak

1 Discipline and punish: the birth of the prison (an excerpt)

Michel Foucault
1975

The following, according to an order published at the end of the seventeenth century, were the measures to be taken when the plague appeared in a town.

First, a strict spatial partitioning: the closing of the town and its outlying districts, a prohibition to leave the town on pain of death, the killing of all stray animals; the division of the town into distinct quarters, each governed by an intendant. Each street is placed under the authority of a syndic, who keeps it under surveillance; if he leaves the street, he will be condemned to death. On the appointed day, everyone is ordered to stay indoors: it is forbidden to leave on pain of death. The syndic himself comes to lock the door of each house from the outside; he takes the key with him and hands it over to the intendant of the quarter; the intendant keeps it until the end of the quarantine. Each family will have made its own provisions; but, for bread and wine, small wooden canals are set up between the street and the interior of the houses, thus allowing each person to receive his ration without communicating with the suppliers and other residents; meat, fish and herbs will be hoisted up into the houses with pulleys and baskets. If it is absolutely necessary to leave the house, it will be done in turn, avoiding any meeting. Only the intendants, syndics and guards will move about the streets and also, between the infected houses, from one corpse to another, the "crows", who can be left to die: these are "people of little substance who carry the sick, bury the dead, clean and do many vile and abject offices". It is a segmented, immobile, frozen space. Each individual is fixed in his place. And, if he moves, he does so at the risk of his life, contagion or punishment.

Inspection functions ceaselessly. The gaze is alert everywhere: "A considerable body of militia, commanded by good officers and men of substance", guards at the gates, at the town hall and in every quarter to ensure the prompt obedience of the people and the most absolute authority of the magistrates, "as also to observe all disorder, theft and extortion". At each of the town gates there will be an observation post; at the end of each street sentinels. Every day, the intendant visits the quarter in his charge, inquires whether the syndics have carried out their tasks, whether the inhabitants have anything to complain of; they "observe their actions". Every day, too, the syndic goes into the street for which he is responsible; stops before each house: gets all the inhabitants to appear at the windows (those who live overlooking the courtyard will be allocated a window looking onto the street at which no one but they may show themselves); he calls each of them by name; informs himself as to the state of each and every one of them "in which respect the inhabitants will be compelled to speak the truth under pain of death"; if someone does not appear at the window, the syndic must ask why: "In this way he will find out easily enough whether dead or sick are being concealed." Everyone locked up in his cage, everyone at his window, answering to his name and showing himself when asked – it is the great review of the living and the dead.

This surveillance is based on a system of permanent registration: reports from the syndics to the intendants, from the intendants to the magistrates or mayor. At the beginning of the "lock up", the role of each of the inhabitants present in the town is laid down, one by one; this document bears "the name, age, sex of everyone, notwithstanding his condition": a copy is sent to the intendant of the quarter, another to the office of the town hall, another to enable the syndic to make his daily roll call. Everything that may be observed during the course of the visits – deaths, illnesses, complaints, irregularities – is noted down and transmitted to the intendants and magistrates. The magistrates have complete control over medical treatment; they have appointed a physician in charge; no other practitioner may treat, no apothecary prepare medicine, no confessor visit a sick person without having received from him a written note "to prevent anyone from concealing and dealing with those sick of the contagion, unknown to the magistrates". The registration of the pathological must be constantly centralized. The relation of each individual to his disease and to his death passes through the representatives of power, the registration they make of it, the decisions they take on it.

Five or six days after the beginning of the quarantine, the process of purifying the houses one by one is begun. All the inhabitants are made to leave; in each room "the furniture and goods" are raised from the ground or suspended from the air; perfume is poured around the room; after carefully sealing the windows, doors and even the keyholes with wax, the perfume is set alight. Finally, the entire house is closed while the perfume is consumed; those who have carried out the work are searched, as they were on entry, "in the presence of the residents of the house, to see that they did not have something on their persons as they left that they did not have on entering". Four hours later, the residents are allowed to re-enter their homes.

This enclosed, segmented space, observed at every point, in which the individuals are inserted in a fixed place, in which the slightest movements are supervised, in which all events are recorded, in which an uninterrupted work of writing links the centre and periphery, in which power is exercised without division, according to a continuous hierarchical figure, in which each individual is constantly located, examined and distributed among the living beings, the sick and the dead – all this constitutes a compact model of the disciplinary mechanism. The plague is met by order; its function is to sort out every possible confusion: that of the disease, which is transmitted when bodies are mixed together; that of the evil, which is increased when fear and death overcome prohibitions. It lays down for each individual his place, his body, his disease and his death, his well-being, by means of an omnipresent and omniscient power that subdivides itself in a regular, uninterrupted way even to the ultimate determination of the individual, of what characterizes him, of what belongs to him, of what happens to him. Against the plague, which is a mixture, discipline brings into play its power, which is one of analysis. A whole literary fiction of the festival grew up around the plague: suspended laws, lifted prohibitions, the frenzy of passing time, bodies mingling together without respect, individuals unmasked, abandoning their statutory identity and the figure under which they had been recognized, allowing a quite different truth to appear. But there was also a political dream of the plague, which was exactly its reverse: not the collective festival, but strict divisions; not laws transgressed, but the penetration of regulation into even the smallest details of everyday life through the mediation of the complete hierarchy that assured the capillary functioning of power; not masks that were put on and taken off, but the assignment to each individual of his "true" name, his "true" place, his "true" body, his "true" disease. The plague as a form, at once real and imaginary, of disorder had as its medical and political correlative discipline. Behind the disciplinary mechanisms can be read the haunting memory of "contagions", of the plague, of rebellions, crimes, vagabondage, desertions, people who appear and disappear, live and die in disorder.

If it is true that the leper gave rise to rituals of exclusion, which to a certain extent provided the model for and general form of the great Confinement, then the plague gave rise to disciplinary projects. Rather than the massive, binary division between one set of people and another, it called for multiple separations, individualizing distributions, an organization in depth of surveillance and control, an intensification and a ramification of power. The leper was caught up in a practice of rejection, of exile-enclosure; he was left to his doom in a mass among which it was useless to differentiate; those sick of the plague were caught up in a meticulous tactical partitioning in which individual differentiations were the constricting effects of a power that multiplied, articulated and subdivided itself; the great confinement on the one hand; the correct training on the other. The leper and his separation; the plague and its segmentations. The first is marked; the second analysed and distributed. The exile of the leper and the arrest of the plague do not bring with them the same political dream. The first is that of a pure community, the second that of a disciplined society. Two ways of exercising power over men, of controlling their relations, of separating out their dangerous mixtures. The plague-stricken town, traversed throughout with hierarchy, surveillance, observation, writing; the town immobilized by the functioning of an extensive power that bears in a distinct way over all individual bodies – this is the utopia of the perfectly governed city. The plague (envisaged as a possibility at least) is the trial in the course of which one may define ideally the exercise of disciplinary power. In order to make rights and laws function according to pure theory, the jurists place themselves in imagination in the state of nature; in order to see perfect disciplines functioning, rulers dreamt of the state of plague. Underlying disciplinary projects the image of the plague stands for all forms of confusion and disorder; just as the image of the leper, cut off from all human contact, underlies projects of exclusion.

2 A viral exception

Jean-Luc Nancy
February 27, 2020

Giorgio Agamben, an old friend, argues that the coronavirus is hardly different from a normal flu (Agamben, 2020). He forgets that for the "normal" flu there is a vaccine that has been proven effective, but even that needs to be readapted to viral mutations year after year. Despite this, the "normal" flu always kills some number of people, while coronavirus, against which there is no vaccine, is evidently capable of causing far higher levels of mortality. The difference (according to sources of the same type as those Agamben uses) is about 1 to 30: it does not seem an insignificant difference to me.

Giorgio states that governments take advantage of all sorts of pretexts to continuously establish states of exception. But he fails to note that the exception is indeed becoming the rule in a world where technical interconnections of all kinds (movement, transfers of every type, impregnation or spread of substances, and so on) are reaching a hitherto unknown intensity that is growing at the same rate as the population. Even in rich countries this increase in population entails a longer life expectancy, hence an increase in the number of elderly people and, in general, of people at risk.

We must be careful not to hit the wrong target: an entire civilization is in question, there is no doubt about it. There is a sort of viral exception – biological, computer-scientific, cultural – which is pandemic. Governments are nothing more than grim executioners, and taking it out on them seems more like a diversionary maneuver than a political reflection.

I mentioned that Giorgio is an old friend. And I apologize for bringing up a personal recollection, but I am not abandoning a register of general reflection by doing so. Almost 30 years ago doctors decided I needed a heart transplant. Giorgio was one of the very few who advised me not to listen to them. If I had followed his advice, I would have probably died soon enough. It is possible to make a mistake. Giorgio is nevertheless a spirit of such finesse and kindness that one may define him – without the slightest irony – as exceptional.

Reference

Agamben, G. (2020, February 26). The invention of an epidemic. *The European Journal of Psychoanalysis*. www.journal-psychoanalysis.eu/coronavirus-and-philosophers/

3 Cured to the bitter end

Roberto Esposito
February 28, 2020

In this text[1] by Nancy I find all the traits that have always characterized him – in particular an intellectual generosity I was personally affected by in the past, drawing immense inspiration from his thinking, especially in my work on communities. What interrupted our dialogue at one point was Nancy's sharp opposition to the paradigm of biopolitics, to which he has always opposed, as in this text, the relevance of technological apparatus – as if the two things were necessarily in contrast. While in fact even the term "viral" itself points to a biopolitical contamination between different languages – political, social, medical and technological – united by the same immune syndrome, meant as a polarity semantically opposed to the lexicon of *communitas*. Though Derrida himself used the category of immunization extensively, Nancy's refusal to confront himself with the paradigm of biopolitics was probably influenced by the dystonia with regard to Foucault that he inherited from Derrida. In any case, we are talking about three of the most important contemporary philosophers.

It remains a fact that anyone with eyes to see cannot deny the constant deployment of biopolitics. From the intervention of biotechnology on domains that were once considered exclusively natural, like birth and death, to bioterrorism, the management of immigration and more or less serious epidemics, all political conflicts today have the relation between politics and biological life at their core. But this reference to Foucault in itself should lead us to not losing sight of the historically differentiated character of biopolitical phenomena. One thing is claiming, as Foucault does, that in the last two and half centuries politics and biology have progressively formed an ever tighter knot, with problematic and sometimes tragic results. Another is to assimilate incomparable incidents and experiences. I would personally avoid making any sort of comparison between maximum-security prisons and a two-week quarantine in the Po lowlands. From the legal point of view, of course, emergency decreeing, long since applied even to cases like this one, in which it is not absolutely necessary, pushes politics towards procedures of exception that may in the long run undermine the balance of power in favor of the executive branch. But to talk of risks to democracy in this case seems to me an exaggeration to say the least. I think that we should try to separate levels and distinguish between long-running processes and recent events. With regard to the former, politics and medicine have been tied in mutual implications for at least three centuries, something that has ultimately transformed both. On the one hand this has led to a process of medicalization of politics, which, seemingly unburdened of any ideological limitations, shows itself as more and more dedicated to "curing" its citizens from risks it is often responsible for highlighting. On the other we witness a politicization of medicine, invested with tasks of social control that do not belong to it, which explains the extremely heterogeneous assessments virologists are making on the nature and gravity of the coronavirus. Both of these tendencies deform politics compared to its classic profile. Also because its objectives no longer comprehend single individuals or social classes, but segments of population differentiated according to health, age, gender or even ethnic group.

But once again, with regard to absolutely legitimate concerns, it is necessary not to lose our sense of proportion. It seems to me that what is happening in Italy today, with the chaotic and rather grotesque overlapping of national and regional prerogatives, has more the character of a breakdown of public authorities than that of a dramatic totalitarian grip.

Note

1 See *A Viral Exception* by Jean-Luc Nancy, https://antinomie.it/index.php/2020/02/27/eccezione-virale/

4   Riposte to Roberto Esposito

Jean-Luc Nancy
February 29, 2020

Dear Robert,

Neither "biology" nor "politics" are precisely determined terms today. I would actually say the contrary. That's why I have no use for their assemblage.

Best regards,
Jean-Luc

5 The community of the forsaken

A response to Agamben and Nancy

Divya Dwivedi and Shaj Mohan
March 8, 2020

India has for long been full of exceptional peoples, making meaningless the notion of "state of exception" or of "extending" it. Brahmins are exceptional, for they alone can command the rituals that run the social order, and they cannot be touched by the lower-caste peoples (let alone desired) for fear of ritualistic pollution. In modern times this involves separate public toilets for them, in some instances. The Dalits, the lowest-caste peoples, also cannot be touched by the upper castes, let alone desired, because they are considered the most "polluting". As we can see, the exception of the Brahmin is unlike the exclusion of the Dalit. One of the Dalit castes named Pariah was turned into a "paradigm" by Arendt, which unfortunately lightened the reality of their suffering. In 1896, when the bubonic plague entered Bombay, the British colonial administration tried to combat the spread of the disease using the Epidemic Diseases Act of 1897. However, caste barriers, including the demand by the upper castes to have separate hospitals and their refusal to receive medical assistance from the lower-caste peoples among the medical personnel, added to causes of the deaths of more than ten million people in India.

The spread of coronavirus,[1] which has infected more than 100,000 people according to official figures, reveals what we wonder about ourselves today: are we worth saving, and at what cost? On the one hand, there are the conspiracy theories which include "bioweapons" and a global project to bring down migration. On the other hand, there are troublesome misunderstandings, including the belief that Covid-19 is something propagated through "corona beer" and the racist commentaries on the Chinese people. But of even greater concern is that, at this conjuncture of the death of god and the birth of mechanical god, we have been persisting in a crisis about the "worth" of man. It can be seen in the responses to the crises of climate, technological "exuberance", and coronavirus.

Earlier, man gained his worth through various *theo-technologies*. For example, one could imagine that the creator and creature were the determinations of something prior, say "being", where the former was *infinite* and the latter *finite*. In such a division, one could think of god as the *infinite man* and man as the *finite god*. In the name of the *infinite man*, the *finite god*s gave the ends to themselves. Today, we are entrusting the machine with the determination of ends, such that its domain can be called *techno-theology*.

It is in this peculiar conjuncture that one must consider Giorgio Agamben's recent remark that the containment measures against Covid-19 are being used as an "exception" to allow an extraordinary expansion of the governmental powers of imposing extraordinary restrictions on our freedoms (Agamben, 2020). That is, the measures taken by most states and at considerable delay, to prevent the spread of a virus that can potentially kill at least 1% of the human population, could implement the next level of "exception". Agamben asks us to choose between "the exception" and the regular while his concern is with the regularization of exception.[2] Jean-Luc Nancy (2000) has since responded to this objection by observing that there are only exceptions today, that is, everything we once considered regular is broken through.[3] Deleuze (1995) in his final text would refer to that which calls to us, at the end of all the games of regularities and exceptions, as "*a life*";[4] that is, one is seized by responsibility when one is confronted with an individual life which is in the seizure of death. *Death and responsibility go together.*

Then let us attend to the non-exceptionality of exceptions. Until the late 1800s, pregnant women admitted in hospitals tended to die in large numbers after giving birth, due to puerperal fever or postpartum infections. At a certain moment, an Austrian physician named Ignaz Semmelweis realized that it was the hands of medical workers carrying pathogens from one autopsy to the next patient, or from one woman's womb to the next, that caused infections and death. The solution proposed by Semmelweis was to wash hands after each contact. For this he was treated as an exception and ostracized by the medical community. He died in a mental asylum suffering from septicemia, which possibly resulted from his being beaten by the guards. Indeed, there are unending senses of exceptions. In Semmelweis's case, the very technique for combating infection was the exception. In *Politics*, Aristotle discussed the case of the exceptional man, such as the one who could sing better than the chorus, who would be ostracized for being a god amongst men.

There is not one paradigm of exception. The pathway of one microbial pathology is different from that of any other. For example, staphylococci live within human bodies without causing any difficulties, although they trigger infections when our immune system response is "excessive". At the extreme of non-pathological relations, the chloroplasts in plant cells and the mitochondria in the cells of our bodies are ancient, well-settled cohabitations between different species. Above all, viruses and bacteria do not "intend" to kill their host, for it is not always in their "interest"[5] to destroy that through which alone they could survive. In the long term – of millions of years of nature's time – "everything learns to live with each other", or at least to obtain equilibria with one another for long periods. This is the biologist's sense of nature's temporality.

In recent years, due in part to farming practices, micro-organisms which used to live apart came together and started exchanging genetic material, sometimes just fragments of DNA and RNA. When these organisms made the "jump" to human beings, disasters sometimes began for us. Our immune systems find these new entrants shocking and then tend to overplay their resources by developing inflammations and fevers which often kill both us *and* the micro-organisms. Etymologically, "virus"[6] is related to poison. It is poison in the sense that by the time a certain new virus finds a negotiated settlement with human animals, we will be long gone. That is, everything can be thought in the model of the "pharmakon" (both poison and cure) if we take nature's time. However, the distinction between medicine and poison in most instances pertains to the time of humans, the uncanny animal. What is termed "biopolitics" takes a stand from the assumption of nature's temporality and thus neglects what is disaster in the view of our interest in – our responsibility for – "a life", that is, the lives of everyone in danger of dying from contracting the virus.

Here lies the crux of the problem: we have been able to determine the "interests" of our immune systems by constituting exceptions in nature, including through the Semmelweis method of handwashing and vaccinations. Our kind of animal does not have biological epochs at its disposal in order to perfect each intervention. Hence, we too, like nature, make coding errors and mutations in nature, responding to each and every exigency in ways we best can. As Nancy noted, man as this technical-exception-maker who is uncanny to himself was thought of very early on by Sophocles in his ode to man. Correspondingly, unlike nature's time, humans are concerned with *this moment*, which must be led to the next moment with the feeling that *we are the forsaken* – those who are cursed to ask after "the why" of their being but without having the means to ask it. Or, as Nancy qualified it in a personal correspondence, "*forsaken by nothing*". The power of this "forsakenness" is unlike the abandonments constituted by the absence of particular things with respect to each other. This forsakenness demands, as we found with Deleuze, that we attend to each life as precious, while knowing at the same time that in the communities of the forsaken we can experience the call of the forsaken individual life which we alone can attend to. Elsewhere, we have called the experience of this call of the forsaken, and the possible emergence of its community from the end of metaphysics and of hypophysics, "anastasis".[7]

Notes

1 Coincidently, the name of the virus "corona" means "crown", the metonymy of sovereignty.
2 Which of course has been perceived as a non-choice by most governments since 2001 in order to securitize all social relations in the name of terrorism. The tendency notable in these cases is that the securitization of the state is proportionate to corporatization of nearly all state functions.
3 See Jean-Luc Nancy (2000).
4 See Gilles Deleuze (1995).
5 It is ridiculous to attribute an interest to a micro-organism, and the clarifications could take much more space than this intervention allows. At the same time, today it is impossible to determine the "interest of man".

6 We should note that "viruses" exist on the critical line between the living and the non-living.
7 In Shaj Mohan and Divya Dwivedi (2019).

References

Agamben, G. (2020, February 26). The invention of an epidemic. *The European Journal of Psychoanalysis*. www.journal-psychoanalysis.eu/coronavirus-and-philosophers/

Deleuze, G. (1995). L'immanence: Une vie [Immanence: A life]. *Philosophie, 47*.

Mohan, S., & Dwivedi, D. (2019). *Gandhi and philosophy: On theological anti-politics* (J. L. Nancy, foreword). Bloomsbury Academic.

Nancy, J. L. (2000). *L'Intrus Galilée* [*The intruder Galileo*]. Bloomsbury Academic.

6   The virtues of the virus

Rocco Ronchi
March 14, 2020

It is difficult to resist the temptation of analogy when trying to make sense of the proportions of the pandemic event. In the reflections that accompany its uncontrolled spread, Covid-19 has become a sort of generalized metaphor, almost the symbolic precipitate of the human condition in post-modernity. What happened 40 years ago with HIV is repeating itself today. The pandemic appears as a sort of *experimentum crucis*, able to test hypotheses that go from politics to the effects of globalization to the transformation of communication at the time of the internet – reaching the heights of the finest metaphysical speculation. The isolation, the mistrust and suspicion the virus causes make it alternatively "populist" and "sovereigntist". The emergency measures it forces upon us seem to universalize the "state of exception" that the present has inherited from the political theology of the twentieth century, confirming Foucault's thesis that modern sovereign power is biopolitical (a power that is articulated in the production, management and administration of "life"). Also, because of the fundamental anonymity characterizing it, the virus seems to share the same immaterial quality that grounds the dominion of financial capitalism. Because of how contagious it is, it can be easily compared to the pre-reflexive and "viral" nature of online communication. Last but not least, the virus signals our eternal human condition. In case we have forgotten that we are mortal, finite, contingent, lacking, ontological, wanting and so forth, the virus is here to remind us, forcing us to meditate and correct our distraction, that of compulsive consumers. These considerations are legitimate. They are, in fact, perfectly justified. This is, however, also their defect. If they make sense, it is precisely because they reduce what is unknown to what is known. They use the virus as intuitive proof that responds – to speak in phenomenological terms – to an expectation that is theoretical. For the critical insight that is being developed around the virus, Covid-19 is rather the name of a science fiction film used to certify previous knowledge.

However, if it is true that the virus displays the characteristic of an event (it would be difficult to deny this), then it must also possess its "virtue". Events are such not because they "happen" or, at least, not only because of this. Events are not "facts". Unlike simple facts, events possess a "virtue", a force, a property, a *vis*, that is, they do something. For this reason, an event is always traumatic to the point we may say that if there is no trauma, there is no event; that if there is no trauma, literally nothing has happened. What exactly do events do? Events produce transformations that prior to their taking place were not even possible. In fact, they only begin to be "after" the event has taken place. In short, an event is such because it generates "real" possibility. One must bear in mind that here "possible" merely means doable. Possibility means being able to do something. Possibility is not something abstract. It is not the free imagination of other worlds that are better than this one. Remaining on a pragmatic level, without indulging in metaphysics, possibility is only "potency" and potency is nothing more than action, determined activity. The "virtue" of an event thus consists in rendering operational methods possible, methods that "before" were simply impossible, unthinkable. It follows that an event can only be thought of starting from the future it generates (and not from the past), because it transforms, because it creates that which is real, and with it possibility. Common sense is therefore right when an event is thought of as an "opportunity" to "make a virtue of necessity".

We are too close to the Covid-19 event to be able to catch a glimpse of the future it bears. Our fear is human, and this makes us unreliable witnesses. However, some signs of the shift in paradigm that this virus is generating are already visible, and they display an unexpected sense. The most striking is probably the sudden disappearance of the ideology linked to "walls". The virus has come at a time when the planet seemed to converge towards the shared belief that the only response to the "threats" posed by globalization consists in redefining guarded borders and strong identities. Populism hates books, but it dogmatically believes in the primacy of "culture", understood in an anthropological sense. The kind of community it promotes is, in fact, historical, romantic and traditional. This community is local by definition, and its sworn enemy is the frigid abstraction of cosmopolitanism. What is even more alien in the eyes of populism is nature, which is nothing other than a resource to be exploited for the well-being of the community (one need only think of Bolsonaro and the deforestation in the Amazon, of Trump and his indifference to global warming, of Salvini's hatred for Greta, etc.). Populists never doubt the idea that humanity is "exceptional". On the contrary, it is an article of faith. I might add that if a populist kisses the cross, it is because this act theologically confirms this exception. In a matter of days, and with an incredible speed, the virus has forced us all, willingly or not, to take upon ourselves – with everyday actions (e.g. wash your hands) – the destiny of the global community and, what is more, the destiny of the community of man with nature. Our culturalist and anthropocentric prejudice was not overcome by the slow and almost always ineffective action of education: a cough was enough to make it suddenly impossible to evade the responsibility that each individual has towards all living beings for the simple fact of (still) being part of this world, and of wanting to be part of it.

With the objective force of trauma, the virus shows that the whole is always implied in the part, that "everything is, in certain sense, in everything" and that in nature there are no autonomous regions that constitute an exception. In nature there is no "dominion within another", as Spinoza wrote, ridiculing the "spirit's" claims to superiority over "matter". The virus's monism is wild and its immanence cruel. If culture de-solidarizes, if it erects barriers and constructs genres, if it defines gradations in the participation in the notion of humanity, tracing horrible borders between "us" and the "barbarians", the virus connects, and forces us to search for common solutions. Nobody, at a time like this, can think it is possible to save oneself on one's own, nor is it possible to do this without involving nature in this process. It is said that the epidemic is leading to the creation of red zones, domestic seclusion and the militarization of territories. This is indeed the case. Here, however, the wall has a completely different meaning compared to the walls the rich build to keep out the poor. A wall is being erected for the other, whoever she or he may be. In times like these, "thy neighbor" is radically reduced to the dimension of "anyone". A wall, in all its forms, including the one meter separating the people standing in bars, is erected to substitute handshakes, now impossible, with that "anyone". It is a means to communicate, not the sign of exclusion. This is confirmed by the fact that the fascist rhetoric has not been able to appropriate these walls and use them to say how right they were about their proposals for segregation. In the face of the immense power of this virus, the fascists have had to put away, at least momentarily, their most effective weapon.

We are too close to the event also to be able to evaluate the effects it will have on the political sphere. There is one fact, however, that must be noted. The virus seems to restore the primacy that once belonged to the political. Classical thought used a metaphor to convey this primacy, the image of a ship's pilot navigating through stormy seas. Thinkers of the past were realists. They knew that there were no safe harbours to enter and end one's journey. Navigation, they said, is necessary, life is not. The "element" washing the political is a kind of nature in which fortune, chance and risk play an ineradicable role. Political "virtue", in fact, consisted in testing the force of this element, governing it with cunning intelligence (*metis*) and resilience. The political is such precisely because it renounces the "human, all too human" illusion that it is possible to appropriate the force of natural elements, an illusion which, on the contrary, constitutes the metaphysical dream of "modern" humanity, which has conceived of the relationship with nature as a war of the spirit against brute matter. Political primacy means governing nature, not dominating it. Also, to explicate the fully "political" nature of this government, it is important to recall the formula so dear to Plato: *kata dynamin*, as much as it is possible for a human. Undoubtedly it is precisely the hypothesis of dominion that is ridiculed by a cough in Wuhan, a cough that makes it necessary to apply the pragmatic intelligence of a ship's pilot to govern, as much as possible, the spontaneity of a process unfolding against our intentions. Covid-19 also possesses this virtue: it commands politics to take on its specific responsibility. It returns the primacy that politics had in delusion left to other sovereign spheres, becoming subordinate to them, declaring its own powerlessness and limiting itself to playing an exclusively technical role. Following Wuhan the agenda can only be set by politics, which must navigate through the stormy seas of a progressive and apparently unstoppable contagion (indeed the Greeks described political virtue as being "cybernetic", that is, nautical). Indeed, what until a few weeks ago seemed to be an unrealistic claim has now become a watchword. Politics must have precedence over the economy. It is the latter that must yield to the needs of the prince, who cares about the destiny of his crew.

Finally, the virus invites us to meditate. I do not think, however, that the object of this meditation is the contingency of being and the precarious nature of human affairs. We certainly do not need Covid-19 to reflect on our fragility. This anxiety has never really disappeared (despite what the journalist in their studios keep saying, when they pontificate about how thanks to the virus humanity, made stupid by the media, so by them, has finally "rediscovered" its ontological insecurity). The virus rather articulates existence, ours and that of others, as "destiny". Suddenly we feel we are being dragged by something that is overpowering, which grows in the silence of our organs, ignoring our will. Is freedom compromised to such an extent? This idea of freedom is certainly mediocre if it conflicts with the inevitability of what takes place. Among the virtues of the virus, we must also mention its ability to generate a more sober idea of freedom: the freedom achieved in doing something about what destiny does to us. To be free is to do what must be done in a specific situation. This is not philosophical abstraction. We see it embodies in the efforts that people make, the earnestness and dedication with which thousands of people work daily to slow the spread of the infection.

Translated from the Italian
by Emma Catherine Gainsforth

7   The threat of contagion

Massimo De Carolis
March 11, 2020

Now that the media storm sparked by the coronavirus is beginning to subside, finally letting some reasonably certain data emerge, while the entire national territory is subjected to a regime of "exceptionality" never experienced before, it is possible to put forward some considerations on how the biological and political spheres are intertwined in the current emergency without fear of confusing the two spheres and thus contributing to the general confusion.

The first fact that appears to be incontestable is the exponential rate with which hospitalizations and deaths increase, doubling in number every two or three days. In short, the epidemic is not an illusion, but a real fact, an epidemic able to bring the hospital system to the brink within a couple of weeks, with dramatic social consequences in regions such as Campania or Sicily, where the health care system is already under strain in normal conditions, for much more futile causes. Conversely, a much more reassuring fact, though not entirely certain, is that the number of people who have contracted the virus with mild symptoms may be much higher than what data shows. In short, it is possible that the virus is less lethal than we originally thought and that the number of infections will start dropping sooner than we think, as positive data from China confirm. It is therefore reasonable to hope that the epidemic will eventually end, without causing millions of deaths the way the Spanish flu or the Asian flu did.

Obviously, hopes are higher because of the greater efficiency of health technologies and systems compared to the past. It is, however, more difficult to measure the effectiveness of the policy measures adopted. The impression is that they are inspired by a principle of common sense. Theoretically, if in Italy no one ever came close to anyone else in the following three weeks (if, absurdly, wives and husbands stopped sleeping together, parents no longer hugged their children and doctors stayed away from patients), it would be impossible for the contagion to spread and the emergency would cease. The government measures seem to aim at this ideal situation as much as possible. Their goal is, if not to cancel social life, at least to suspend it until further notice, relying on remote technology such as social networks and smart working for communication. The reasoning behind these measures, whether it is right or wrong, appears to be shared by the vast majority of the population, which is adapting to the new rules with surprising zeal. Certainly not everyone thinks that kids gathering to celebrate a birthday, or that the elderly who insist on having a coffee in a bar, despite these measures, are irresponsible "criminals". But certainly, at the moment, obedience to the rules is strengthened by strong social disapproval of the offenders. Therefore, demanding the mitigation or even a suspension of these measures would be, at the moment, a futile and unpopular move, especially since no one seems to have a viable alternative.

The fact remains, however, that these measures are disturbing. They dissolve the social bond and impose a regime of loneliness and police control on the whole population, a strong reminder of the darkest experiences of our recent political past. The crucial point is therefore to understand whether this is really and *only* a simple parenthesis, or if we are rather witnessing a general test of what could become the condition of ordinary life in the societies of the near future.

This doubt is justified by the fact that the destruction of the social bond and obsessive control in the name of "public health" certainly did not originate with the coronavirus. For at least a century, modern social mechanisms have tended to generate a society based on isolation, in which the spontaneity of social life is perceived as an obstacle or even a threat to the stability of the system. The point is that in the past the production system could not function without bodies, voices and hands working together: it could limit and control promiscuity but not eliminate it entirely. Today, on the contrary, all of this is possible, thanks to the wonders of technology. For the first time, despite how paradoxical this may sound, the machine reproducing society can completely eliminate human sociality, without paying too high a price. What guarantees that this is not what is being tested for the future?

To avoid misunderstandings, let us make it clear that in no case will a conspiracy, a Spectre or some more or less occult personification of Power correspond to this question. There is no director behind social phenomena. These are the result of a varying number of independent forces and drives. There are no puppeteers, only puppets animating the theatre, each in his or her own way, with more or less force, in one direction or another, often in spite of their conscious intentions. When the epidemic is over, there will certainly be a festive return to sociality, which no democratic government will dream of prohibiting. Certainly, however, many companies will decide that smart working is convenient and will ask employees not to dismantle the emergency workstations they have arranged in their bedrooms. Many conformist people will notice that the closure of nightlife venues is an advantage for public safety, provided it does not harm the interests of restaurants and tourism. Also, many "identitarian" political forces will remind us that contagion, in general, spreads among homeless people and immigrants in particular (although exceptionally not in this case), and that the public health system requires unyielding hygiene. More generally, all of us will discover that, ultimately, there is no social life that does not involve risk of contagion, just as there is no organic life that does not involve the risk of disease and death. For this reason we will have to address a basic political question: to what extent are we willing to jeopardize, also minimally, our biological security to have dinner with a friend, to embrace a child or simply to chat with the people hanging around in the square? Where do we place the bar when deciding that our social happiness has precedence over safeguarding our health? Is political existence more important than biological survival?

The fact that the coronavirus is forcing us to ask these questions from one day to the next is a good thing, because the structure of our future society may depend on the answers we provide *with facts* (not only words).

**Translated from the Italian
by Emma Catherine Gainsforth**

8   What carries us on

Shaj Mohan
March 23, 2020

Implicit within the debate on coronavirus curated by *Antinomie* and archived by the *European Journal of Psychoanalysis*[1] is the question *for what must we carry on?* That is, do we – humanity, which has been reckoned by many thinkers as the error in nature – carry on for the sake of carrying on? Or, should we, following Thomas Taylor, M. K. Gandhi, Pierre Clastres, and several others, proceed with a project of returning towards a moment in history that, for Agamben (2020), is "the normal conditions of life"? Is not Agamben's notion of normal life none other than a mythical European bourgeois idyll where "the churches" do not "remain silent"? Should we continue to evaluate everything in our present with these "normal conditions of life"?

These conversations have been happening in America, too, where "the boomers" – those few of a post-war generation who enjoyed prosperity and *relatively stable* conditions of life – evaluate the lives of "millennials" on the basis of their own myths and idylls. Wittgenstein distinguished the philosopher from the bourgeois thinker who thinks "with the aim of clearing up the affairs of some particular community". It is impossible to avoid the fact that the "normal conditions of life" to be guarded from "biopolitics" were, and are, dependent on colonial, capitalistic, and other exploitative processes which all these families of thoughts including the theory of "biopolitics" seek to criticize. Since the notions of "normalcy" and "biopolitics" held by Agamben, and derived from Michel Foucault, have been exported through analogy over regions of the world and of thought that are homologically distinct, a certain "bourgeois thinking" has become the universal today. In many parts of the world these theories provide the experience of a conspiratorial spirit in history determining its course, leaving humans to merely lament, which is our sense of "resistance" today.

The terror before this question – *for what must we carry on?* – was always understood and it is not limited to any epoch or region. The closing off of this question has been mostly the work of what we call "religions". However, it began to acquire an urgency with Nietzsche's destruction of all values towards a revaluation of all values. Nietzsche pointed to an obscure object of thought as the reference for the revaluation of all values – *eternal return of the same.* Martin Heidegger would execute a certain act in philosophy in 1934 which would then suppress the import of the question *for what must we carry on?* in a lecture course titled "Logic as the Question Concerning the Essence of Language". In this lecture, long before Foucault and Agamben, Heidegger specified a certain form of politics – "population politics" – which considers people with indifference to their bloodlines and 'tongue-lines'. He wrote:

> In a census, the *Volk* is counted in the sense of the population, the population, in so far as it constitutes the body of the *Volk*, the inhabitants of the land. At the same time, it is to be considered that in a governmental *order* of the census a certain part of the *Volk* is included, namely the part that dwells within the State's borders. The German nationals living abroad are not included in the count, [they] do not belong in this sense to the *Volk*. On the other hand, those can also be included in the count, *those who, taken racially, are of alien breed, do not belong to the Volk.*
>
> (Heidegger, 2009, p. 56)

Here, population refers to something of a "motley crew", whereas the ideal type for "a people" are those dwellers of the soil who once enjoyed a mythic unity with one another. Here is a German bourgeois thinker.

If we assume that this tendency of the last century is "Eurocentric", it will be a grave error. In fact, its most profound and startling expression can be found in the subcontinent. M. K. Gandhi too conceived an Indian village idyll and contrasted it with "western civilization". Gandhi's idyll is the village of the privileged upper-caste Indian under whom the racial hierarchies and exploitations of the majority lower-caste people carry on, but without an ounce of resentment on the part of the exploited. The logic of surrendering to the caste order without resentment in the subcontinent is called "Karman" (Agamben, 2018). Gandhi understood that this ideal was never realized in history, and never will be.

However, Gandhi's evaluation of mankind was not founded on the ideal village as the "normal conditions". Instead, the village itself was founded on the principles of hypophysics, according to which nature is the good. We had called this mode of thinking hypophysics following Kant's taxonomy of moral thought (Mohan & Dwivedi, 2019). The ideal Indian village is the home of hypophysics where all things are retained at their original value, that is, a place where nature was never de-natured. The ideal village conserves the "normal conditions" in spite of the presence of Man. Gandhi's verdict was that Man was infected with a range of faculties that allowed him to explore all the milieus given in nature and also propelled him to discover the milieus unknown to nature. The being without an appropriate milieu is the effervescent error in nature. If a being cannot be given a fixed milieu, then what is good and bad for it are also indefinable. That is, action in the moral sense is impossible for such a being, who must therefore seek its own dissolution in nature.

As we know, Gandhi's goal in life was to reduce himself to "zero", a point at which no action was required. As with all rigorous thinkers, he sought the same end for humankind itself – *we must not carry on*. Gandhi's advice to Martin Buber on the fate of the Jewish people in Nazi Germany came from his interpretation of "for what must we carry on". When Gandhi was requested by Buber to intervene on behalf of the Jewish people using his considerable moral standing in the world, he responded:

> The calculated violence of Hitler may even result in a general massacre of the Jews by way of his first answer to the declaration of such hostilities. But if the Jewish mind could be prepared for voluntary suffering, even the massacre I have imagined could be turned into a day of thanksgiving and joy that Jehovah had wrought *deliverance of the race* even at the hands of the tyrant. For to the godfearing, death has no terror.
>
> (Gandhi, 2006, p. 420)

The schema of this response, shocking as it is, continues to reign over our time. What holds the schema together is hypophysics, and the theory of "biopolitics" is itself a species of hypophysics.

Today, the dominance of this tendency – hypophysics – is not to be scorned upon without understanding the conditions in which it arose. Hypophysics came to be dominant when metaphysics became impossible; that is, instead of referring to another domain for values we began to find the Ideal within our preferred socio-economic milieus and in the calamitous misunderstandings of nature. We became acutely aware of the absence of "value" and hence a certain inability to distinguish between good and evil in the last century. We must note that this aversion of the eye from the absence of value, which makes one hold fast to the nearest ideal or idyll, is still a caring thought.

The formalization of the experience of being without value, without an orientation in the face of the question *for what must we carry on?*, is most acutely found in the schema of Heidegger's early works.[2] In philosophy, difference is found in something which is differentiable. For example, we say that "1" and "a" differ in the differentiable "written characters". Duns Scotus's theology relies on thinking being as the ultimate differentiable in which God was the infinite being and creatures the finite beings. This gives us something akin to *infinite man* and *finite gods* to work with. Being, in which the difference is made, gives man his orientation in God. The similarity between the logic of this division in being and the theory of Idea in Plato's middle period made Nietzsche remark that Christianity was Platonism for the masses.

Heidegger would propose a new kind of difference without precedence – ontico-ontological difference or the difference between *being* and *beings* – for which there is no differentiable. From this moment, being could not be thought as something that is the primary differentiable, nor could it be thought as the place holder for the higher beings – Idea, Subject, Will – for there is no primary differentiable. Heidegger's unthinkable logic would open the mystery of being itself and at the same time keep in abeyance the unthinkable through the narrative of the decline in the history of the difference between being and beings. In this narrative, there once was an ideal village in Greece where "normal conditions of living" were available.

Jean-Luc Nancy (1997) pursued and revealed the limits of this thought when he wrote the obscure proposition *"existence precedes and succeeds upon itself"* (p. 34). It stands outside the family of propositions such as "existence precedes essence" and "essence precedes existence", and it implies at least two things. First, reason can be given for the succession of each thing upon itself and of a thing upon another thing. However, there is no reason, under any other names, for the persistence of existence. Second, we can determine our actions, or our movement from moment to moment, through reason which drives this movement in spite of us. However, we are abandoned in the face of the moment itself, which does not submit to reason. That is, the *duratio noumenon* is properly obscure. The world wraps around us with its intrigues of reason while at the same time reason itself drives us towards the absence of itself in the fact of reason, a seizure from which one cannot shake free.

In a series of proper names – Wittgenstein, Heidegger, Derrida, Deleuze, Nancy – and through different logics and systematicities, we have come to an acute understanding of this fact: that we are *forsaken*. But what does it imply, especially now when we are seeking an orientation in the face of an epidemic and then other calamities? In a short text with the least formal steps, something can still be indicated and shared. Anticipation is when we say that "there is lighting, and thunder is set to follow". When several elements are involved in the constitution of a phenomenon our anticipations are likely to meet with disappointment or surprise; for example, a concert may be cancelled due to an earthquake. The moments, and the relation between the moments, which we can account for through reason can fall within the experience of anticipation; that is, everything in the world. However, there is something outside anticipation – the persistence of the world – which we embrace with the absolute certainty that its disappearance with us in it is never a concern, although we know that "a world" of a "someone" will withdraw, including our own. In each step of anticipations and disappointments we are surprised by this disorienting certitude. If we bring Kant and Wittgenstein together, *the end of the world is not an event, for it is not an event in the world.*

This absolute certitude is the most obscure experience, while also being the most distinct. Like a membrane, it envelops everything while penetrating everything as we look into everything. Early Wittgenstein's experience of this mystery was that of the individual who in his solitude experienced the sense of the world lying outside it while the being of the world itself was for that very reason obscure. But what we can say, for now, is that this experience of the obscure – the assurance of an absolute persistence – is possible on the condition that we are able to speak with one another in sharing our reasons and responsibilities. Later Wittgenstein would argue that the possibility of each experience is public, for there is no private language. Then, each one of us, without knowing the whence and whither of it, share the obscure because we can share words, cultures, love, cautions and tragedies.

From the experience of the obscure we should think of the other side of hypophysics, which is technological determinism. It is the same aversion from the obscure experience that turns us towards technological exuberance where a new god is being founded – the hyper-machines that will make machines which humans can neither build nor comprehend. It will be these machines that will then give ends to man. Biopolitics and other theories are rendering us immobile and resigned like animals who are caught in the headlights, but of our own rushing technical exuberance.

Tonight we should rest a while in our shared solitude (the only kind of solitude as we can see) with the thought that the mystery is not that the world is, but that it is mysterious to us *making of us the mystery*, the obscure *mysterium tremendum*. In the words of the poet, tonight we are *"Alive in the Superunknown"*.

Notes

1 See Coronavirus and Philosophers. www.journal-psychoanalysis.eu/coronavirus-and-philosophers/; https://antinomie.it
2 Wittgenstein's *Tractatus Logico-philosophicus* (1922) arrived at the absence of any kind of "for what" for us to "carry on" before Heidegger came into the scene, but it did so through a different logic.

References

Agamben, G. (2018). *Karman: A brief treatise on action, guilt, and gesture*. Stanford University Press.
Agamben, G. (2020). The enemy is not outside, it is within us. *The Bookhaven*. http://bookhaven.stanford.edu/2020/03/giorgio-agamben-on-coronavirus-the-enemy-is-not-outside-it-is-within-us/
Gandhi, R. (2006). *Gandhi: The man, his people, and the empire*. University of California Press.
Heidegger, M. (2009). *Logic as the question concerning the essence of language*. SUNY Press.
Mohan, S., & Dwivedi, D. (2019). *Gandhi and philosophy: On theological anti-politics*. Bloomsbury Academic.
Nancy, J. L. (1997). *Sense of the world*. University of Minnesota Press.
Wittgenstein, L. (1922). *Tractatus logico-philosophicus*. Routledge.

9   The obscure experience

Shaj Mohan
April 13, 2020

Implicitly, what we are asking in these discussions about the Covid-19 pandemic[1] is a familiar question: *is there a norm for man?* Earlier it was philosophy that had the task of constituting the systems under which the limits, and also the as yet unknown thresholds, for actions were given. Aristotle wrote in *The Politics*:

> A ship which is only a span long will not be a ship at all, nor a ship a quarter of a mile long; yet there may be a ship of a certain size, either too large or too small, which will still be a ship, but bad for sailing.
>
> (1984, 1326b1, Book 7)

In the same text, Aristotle set the criteria for cities, especially the ideal distance between the well-governed city and the seas. It would appear that the further the seas, the better. Even today, the threat posed by the sea is of the unfamiliar, the obscure, the strangers, the refugees and the degenerates. For these very reasons which provoke distaste in most of us today, the criteria of the Greek cartel with a constitution, run by a few men and excluding women and slaves from their "democracy", cannot be our criteria for politics.

We assume from the common uses of the terms "natural" and "normal" that nature is a set of norms. A principle of this misleading thought is Spinoza's *conatus* – the tendency in all beings to conserve in their own being. However, if there is a tendency in everything (in so far as things are), it is to prolong itself sufficiently in a "milieu" in order to enjoy being-other-than-oneself, and to be elsewhere. These changes vary in their temporalities across living systems and within each living system. Most cells in our body renew themselves in weeks, immunities are acquired, and mutations are undergone. Homeostasis refers to the relative stability as a "species" characteristic,[2] while speciation exchanges a previous set of powers for a new set of powers. Darwin was concerned with the ratio holding between the external and internal milieus of living forms; we can understand it as the reciprocal adjustment of internal and external forms. *Nature is hardly normal.* That is, form in living form is not Platonic form, but it is something akin to the clinch of the wrestlers appearing to be indistinguishable from a tight embrace.

The being which is challenging us, the virus, is somewhere between our concept of the living and the non-living. Guido Pontecorvo, the geneticist born in Pisa, made certain predictions about viral pandemics in 1948, suggesting that two non-virulent forms of viruses infecting the same host may produce a new form which will then result in pandemics of the type we are undergoing. The idea underlying this prediction was that viruses sexually reproduce, which violates our most familiar "norm" of life. The "normalized" concept of sexual reproduction involves the presence of specialized organs for the exchange of genetic material. But in fact, any mechanism through which genetic recombination takes place is sexual reproduction.[3]

We have been, especially in recent years, attributing norms to ourselves and to what is called nature. These attributions have a general principle – *hypophysics* – which takes nature to coincide with the good: a thing is good when it is proximate to its nature, and is evil when it departs from that nature. The moralization of the earth system and of animals today is easily recognizable. Norms have been prescribed for the human animal as well. For example, "normal conditions of life" as that which is natural to man and from which every deviation is viewed with suspicion. While metaphysics withdrew from the task of providing the grounds upon which norms could be laid out and given to man, a proliferation of hypophysical schemas appeared alongside it. The thinkers of these schemas were diverse in their styles and their choice of domains – Thomas Taylor, M. K. Gandhi, Jacques Ellul, Pierre Clastres, Giorgio Agamben.

In this series of thinkers, Pierre Clastres stands out, for he too had a norm, albeit not of his own milieu but of what he called "primitive society". The deviation from the norm in a primitive society makes "the state" appear, and this is the very instant in which Man is de-natured. Clastres sought the archeology of the state in primitive societies. But all he could find was that when something, such as a metal axe, enters the primitive society from the outside (the modern world) their *conatus* collapses. We must see in his own words the perfect picture of human norm, or conatus: "Primitive society, then, is a society from which nothing escapes, which lets nothing get outside itself, for all the exits are blocked. *It is a society, therefore, that ought to reproduce itself perpetually without anything affecting it throughout time*" (Clastres, 2007, p. 212).

Let us call the theories of all these proposed norms *idyllic a priori*, following from the example set by Foucault. Idyllic a priori are derivative of hypophysics; that is, a moment in the history of a few is interpreted as the natural way of being because this is the "normal conditions of life" for them. Behind the many theories of "biopolitics" lie their respective idyllic a priori.

A series of philosophical works in the last century, which can be recalled through the names of concepts – logical form, *Destruktion*, deconstruction, difference, existence – and the names of philosophers – Wittgenstein, Heidegger, Deleuze, Derrida, Nancy – showed us that the conditions for determining norms were not with us anymore.[4] We found through these tumultuous days of thinking that *nature is not natural*. And yet, we retain a certain relation with reason: we assume that each and everything befalls us not without reason, rather everything drives us to give them reason. We know that we can anticipate the coursing of one thing into the next, or the transition from one state to the next. Even this pandemic was anticipated several times in the past. When the anticipation meets with the objective there is satisfaction; for example, every August we anticipate the Perseid meteor shower and it does not disappoint us. When anticipation is not satisfied in experience, there is either surprise or disappointment. In spite of all the anticipations regarding various calamities of the world, we proceed with an absolute certainty that this world itself will not withdraw, that it will not disappoint, although we cannot give a reason for it, for there is no reason[5] why it should not withdraw in this very instant. Reason drives us towards this experience just as we are drawn to it. Logically we can accommodate this experience – which is the most shared and even mundane experience of humankind – by saying that *the end of the world is not an event in the world, and therefore it is not an event.*[6] For now, let us mark it as *the obscure experience.* Today we are left with this shared mundane mystery which cannot be encoded in reason, although it surrounds reason. This commonplace experience – the absolute certitude that the world will persist – does not institute any norm, for it is obscure. Instead, it makes a demand that we do not "play" politics in such a way that it – the most shared of all experiences – is surrendered either to an idyllic a priori or to technological exuberance.

It is time to think again of our relation to technology, both bio-techniques and computational techniques, and their growing proximity. Some radical shifts in our humankind began in the 19th century when Simmelweis introduced through the technique of hand washing as a barrier between us and microbes. Further, through Koch, Pasture and several others we began to take charge of our "immune systems" and direct them according to our interests using vaccines, antivirals and immunosuppressive medicines. The emergent nano-machines (atomic scale engineering is already a reality; Frei et al., 2019) will course through our circulatory system such that our immune systems will be completely externalized. This will complete our new "speciation".

We are also the species that drew a circulatory system upon the earth. When "we" began to wander the earth, nearly 50,000 years ago, we had already begun the processes of inter-connecting the regions of the earth, which resulted in the Silk Road and the internet. There are many instances in which we can see that the externalized immune system and the global circulatory system of internet and commodities are conjoined. For example, the very medicines which regulate the immune system are produced in Asia and then travel to the rest of the world. Bio-medical systems can be remotely managed through the internet. Together we are coming to be a singular organism of our own making on earth.

Then what of the earth? Although it might seem an abhorrent thought, "the earth" too is already implicated in this circulatory system, which began at least with agriculture. The global circulatory system will suffer the traumas of the two kinds of viral infections again. As Mohammed and Sandberg (2020) argue, the virulence of both the computer virus and the organic virus will be a function of the rate of integration of the global circulatory system, and they show that the organic virus too will soon be engineered.[7]

Today, nationalisms and various ethno-centric proclivities stand in the way of the well-being of the global circulatory system. Due to potential bio-cyber wars between nation states the global circulatory system itself is under threat. Eventually the components of these older orders of the world will be comprehended by a new set of laws. However, now is the time and the occasion (when this flu is being experienced in the global circulatory system) for us to think together about the future forms of our being together as those who are shared by the commonplace and yet obscure experience. This way we return to the beginning: unless we as everyone, everywhere, understand that this world is the co-belonging equally of everyone in sharing the mysterious but absolute certainty of its persistence, and create political concepts and new institutions, this ship might become either too small or too large to set sail ever again.

Notes

1 See www.journal-psychoanalysis.eu/coronavirus-and-philosophers/
2 The concept of "subspecies" appeared as unhelpful in the textbooks of evolutionary biology decades ago. Today "species" is being thought without the scholastic exactness. The concept of "milieu" too has undergone revisions and biologists do not practice with "milieu" as something which is "fixed".
3 See Bernstein et al. (1984).
4 Metaphysics fixed norms by taking "being" as the fundamental differentiable. The differentiated are not predicable of the differentiable; that is, we never say that "function is a linear equation." In metaphysics these operations created a series of differences such as that between Idea and things, God and creatures, and so on. Of these pairs the first term is the higher being which then grounds the norms for man. Heidegger would produce a remarkable new division, that between being and beings, which is without a differentiable, and would call it ontico-ontological difference. This strange difference – if it makes sense, it is not understood – brought metaphysics to a point of suspension. See Mohan (2020; see also Chapter 8 in this volume).
5 In the restricted use of reason.
6 This thought can only be suggested here. For more, see "What Carries Us On" in www. journal-psychoanalysis.eu/coronavirus-and-philosophers/ and https://antinomie.it/
7 Working paper titled "Hybrid Risk: Cyber-Bio Risks," shared kindly by Anish Mohammed and Anders Sandberg.

References

Aristotle. (1984). *The complete works of Aristotle* (J. Barnes, Ed.). Princeton University Press.
Bernstein, H., Byerly, H. C., Hopf, F. A., & Michod, R. E. (1984, October 7). Origin of sex. *Journal of Theoretical Biology, 110*(3), 323–351.
Clastres, P. (2007). *Society against the state* (R. Hurley, Trans., reprint). Zone Books.
Frei, M. S., Mondelli, C., García-Muelas, R., Kley, K. S., Puértolas, B., López, N., Safonova, O. V., Stewart, J. A., Ferré, D. C., & Pérez-Ramírez, J. (2019). Atomic-scale engineering of indium oxide promotion by palladium for methanol production via CO2 hydrogenation. *Nature Communications, 10*, 3377.

Mohammed, A., & Sandberg, A. (2020). *Hybrid risk: Cyber-bio risks* (Working Paper). Routledge.

Mohan, S. (2020). What carries us on. *European Journal of Psychoanalysis.* www.journal-psychoanalysis.eu/coronavirus-and-philosophers/; https://antinomie.it/www.nature.com/articles/s41467-019-11349-9

10 Agamben, the virus, and the biopolitical

A riposte

Zsuzsa Baross
April 17, 2020

During the early phase of the epidemic, Agamben published a series of provocative statements in the media, charging that:

> our society no longer believes in anything but bare life. It is obvious that Italians are disposed to sacrifice practically everything – the normal conditions of life, social relationships, work, even friendships, affections and religious and political convictions – to the danger of getting sick. Bare life – and the danger of losing it – is not something that unites people, but blinds and separates them.
>
> (Agamben, 2020a)

★ ★ ★

The mistake, or shall I say after Deleuze, the *bêtise*, of Agamben's response[1] to the new coronavirus ("the invention of an epidemic") is not that it mistakes the pathogen for a "normal" flu – an infection whose victims are small in number and, for the most part, with light or moderate symptoms (even though by late February when the first provocative piece appeared,[2] the scale of the devastation in Wuhan and elsewhere was evident, whether or not it constituted an "event" [that Agamben invites us to reread François Brune's *Ces évènements qui n'existent pas* implies that the answer to this question should be negative]; besides the question of competence, the category "normal" has a questionable place in virology, as the history of epidemics, as the devastation of the natives of the Americas attest; viruses "normalize" or/ and get "normalized.").

But Agamben (2020b), as he will remind his critics in a later interview, is not an epidemiologist or virologist; he does not intervene in the question in the capacity of a specialist in infectious diseases. The error (this time neither mistake nor *bêtise*) concerns not the nature of the virus itself (which is Nancy's argument) but lies at the very heart of his philosophical project and its application/invocation of the (old) concept of the biopolitical (and the state of exception as its purest form) with regard to the time of the day, today: the time of the "geocide" (Michel Deguy), the climate "collapse," the generalized catastrophe (collapse of coordinates). The flaw in the argument that the fear of the manufactured epidemic is (put) in the service of the political (governments) and responds to the real need for a collective panic – for which the "epidemic is an ideal pretext" – is not that it underestimates the force or potency of the epidemic for (biological, economic, social, cultural) devastation (which it does); nor does it lie in reading the aggressive governmental responses to the epidemic as essentially and fundamentally "biopolitical"; rather, it lies in failing to grasp these responses as manifestations and symptoms of a radical mutation in the field: the inversion of the *order* of the articulation *bio/political*, the *détournement* and reversal of the direction of forces that traverse the nexus which inexorably, irrevocably, and today without mercy, binds *bios* (organic and inorganic life) to the political.

The "biopolitical"

As we know, Agamben's re-appropriation of Foucault's concept turns the biopolitical into an axiomatic "thesis": the political (of the West) is always already biopolitical, is constituted as such, as the exclusion (fabrication) of "bare life" at the point of its origin (Aristotle, the Greeks). I leave aside here my reservation regarding this initial founding gesture and recall only that Arendt's reading of the same history generates a different structure and narrative of the origin. It assigns the creation of the political – the founding distinction/division (*oikos/polis*; *zoe/bios*) – to the performative work of the Law that belongs to neither domain (Arendt, 1958). The Law (or the Wall, the physical manifestation of the nomos) orders the city it constitutes into two distinct spaces it itself separates: *oikos*, or the private space of "privation" (production/reproduction // need and necessity // birth and death), and *polis*, or the public space of visibility, exposure, action. True, the *polis* excludes *zoe* from its domain: the "metabolism of life" is hidden from view on the other side of the Wall by the Wall. But the Wall, this early precursor of "separation," unlike the contemporary variety that creates enclaves, only separates, sorts out, makes a categorical distinction; the Greek citizen, the citizen-body, crosses over the Wall daily and is the habitant of both domains. In other words, the *polis* excludes but does not capture, hold captive what it excludes. The structure, *oikos/polis*, in this Arendtian rendition, is irreducibly heterogeneous to the "inclusive exclusion" yet to come in the future, whose "paradigm is the camp," which in turn is the "nomos of the modern" (Agamben, 1998).

One need not embrace Arendt's narrative reconstruction of the origin to see the slippage (perhaps even sleight of hand) in Agamben regarding Foucault's biopolitical. The "always already" smooths over, flattens out the disruptive gesture of Foucault's genealogy, which cuts into the flow of history, inserting into it the discontinuity of a heterogenizing mutation; namely, a new political or governmentality that, unlike the sovereign power it replaces, takes charge of life (Foucault, 1990). In Agamben's revision, the Foucauldian genealogy of heterogeneous formations is contracted, its discontinuity replaced by a long and continuous biopolitical history and "development" (I use his term with caution as a shorthand) which, while filled with repetitions, resemblances, precursors, forgotten originals, and returns, is still, in the last instance, always the biopolitical fabrication of bare life. In its purest, that is, its most reductive form, the biopolitical becomes the state of exception – the most reductive form and absolute limit case with regard to both life and, paradoxically, the political itself, for absolute power over absolutely reduced life is achieved at the cost of the Law rendering itself inoperative, by law. "It encompasses living beings by means of its own [lawful] suspension" (Agamben, 1998).

We can see how the emergencies recently declared all over the world would lead or permit Agamben (2020c) to recognize in them the classical *form* of the state of exception, now normalized:

> What is once again manifest is the tendency to use a state of exception as a normal paradigm for government. The legislative decree immediately approved by the government "for hygiene and public safety reasons" actually produces an authentic militarization of the municipalities and areas with the presence of at least one person who tests positive and for whom the source of transmission is unknown, or in which there is at least one case that is not ascribable to a person who recently returned from an area already affected by the virus. Such a vague and undetermined definition will make it possible to rapidly extend the state of exception to all regions, as it's almost impossible that other such cases will not appear elsewhere. Let's consider the serious limitations of freedom the decree contains: a) a prohibition against any individuals leaving the affected municipality or area; b) a prohibition against anyone from outside accessing the affected municipality or area; c) the suspension of events or initiatives of any nature and of any form of gatherings in public or private places, including those of a cultural, recreational, sporting and religious nature, including enclosed spaces if they are open to the public; d) the closure of kindergartens, childcare services and schools of all levels, as well as the attendance of school, higher education activities and professional courses, except for distance learning; e) the closure to the public of museums and other cultural institutions and spaces as listed in article 101 of the code of cultural and landscape heritage, pursuant to Legislative Decree 22 January 2004, no. 42. All regulations on free access to those institutions and spaces are also suspended; f) suspension of all educational trips both in Italy and abroad; g) suspension of all public examination procedures and all activities of public offices, without prejudice to the provision of essential and public utility services; h) the enforcement of quarantine measures and active surveillance of individuals who have had close contacts with confirmed cases of infection.

★ ★ ★

Whether at the point of its origin or, for Agamben (2005), in its purest state, the state of exception, or again, in its latest variety of bio-economico-political order, power always flows from the political in the direction of life: toward its regulation, control, dressage, confinement; its manipulation, exploitation, putting it to work (see insulin production), turning it to a weapon (biological warfare); or as power becomes ever more creative, it moves towards recombination (DNA), transplantation, hybridization, manufacture – and, in the last instance, not in terms of chronology, the fabrication of life as bare life.

The state of exception therefore is also exceptional in this regard: it targets to control the whole of life.

As structure, perhaps, but certainly as (empty) *form*, the state of exception would appear to cover – as a lid covers what falls under it – the multiple ever more draconian, ever more restrictive regulations recently enacted: distancing, spacing, quarantine, confinement, self-isolation, and most recently, the tracking of movements and contacts of bodies – citizen bodies.

And yet, something escapes. First, the virus escapes. Literally. From the rainforest of the Democratic Republic of the Congo, from the wild (wildlife: bat, pangolin [a rare anteater]) in Wuhan, a life form escapes, an RNA sequence that is not even properly alive. It leaps over the barrier between species, escapes its confinement to "nature", its assigned proper (own) territory. Following, opportunistically exploiting the routes and pathways of globalization – that other aggressive, indiscriminate invader – it itself globalizes, but englobes not the globe or the earth, but the World.[3] In Jean-Luc Nancy's terminology: space(s) where sense circulates. In Deleuze's language, it deterritorializes from "nature," the "wild" (or the bio-lab), and simultaneously reterritorializes (there is no deterritorialization without reterritorialization) the "socio-political domain"; it leaps over to the other side of the Wall of separation that long ago constituted its territory by confining it on the inside. In other words, the direction of invasion, intervention, penetration – that is, of forces passing though the nexus – gets reversed: now they flow from the direction of life; the *sense* (in every sense of this word) of the biopolitical gets inverted as it is the political body/the body of the political that is invaded, attacked. The tissue of connections that make and remake this body is torn apart, in self-defense; the biological, living citizen body is forced to retreat from public spaces, to take refuge in the space of privation, the *oikos*, leaving the virus to circulate in the public space, more or less freely. (And not just the virus: as we learnt recently, wild animals, foxes and coyotes have been returning to the streets of the city. In South Africa, a pride of lions has been photographed sleeping lazily on an empty highway.) The state of exception (if this term still applies) in the case of this "novel" virus is not the exercise of power over life as bare life but, on the contrary, an extreme (exceptional) self-defensive measure and immune reaction by the political body to an invading life form that is not even properly alive.

The biopolitical: we have been so certain, so confident of our control over our own "invention" (as Agamben understands this term, as a political construction), "nature," as distinct and separate, a domain apart, that our lan-guage left out the hyphen that would mark the conjunction, designating the place of articulation where forces cross over, and which is also the weakest point in the construction, opening up the *concept* to deconstruction on the one hand, and the political, the life and the only life our societies have known for some time, to a potentially total destruction on the other. The notion (again Agamben's) that the "contagion" would be an invention of the political is thus a fantasy that belongs to this same old biopolitical order, without a hyphen, whose order (ordering of the relation) has been overturned, whose forces (first "containment," then "mitigation") have been, to stay with the war metaphors so popular nowadays, de-routed and, so far, defeated. Not just by the newly discovered, infinitely inventive virus, but by the far more massive and irrevers-ible contagion that will not go away when "all this ends," and has been on course for some time: the climate catastrophe, collapse or geocide, which is the terrain on which this epidemic unfolds, their common "transmitter" being, as we well know, globalization.

The biopolitical response to the contagion, a state of exception, is thus a defensive immune reaction, or more precisely, a reaction of auto-immunity (in Derrida's precise definition of this term) that turns against the very body it is designed to defend. It acts into, destroys the connective tissue of the political body: it interrupts the flow of communication, closes border crossings, isolates, prohibits contact, confines, excludes, isolates; it punctuates public spaces by opening up gaps, inserting intervals; it empties cinemas and theaters, turns the grand boulevards of great cities into deserts, commands a distance large enough between bodies to prevent contact even by the air exhaled. (In its mechanism of auto-defense, the political thus mimics the living body, whose excessive immune reaction to the virus destroys the body itself: it floods the lungs and, depriving it of oxygen, brings about its total organ failure.)

"Bare life" vs. "*a* life"

A personal digression is perhaps permissible at the time of this pandemic: for days the phrase or syntagma "born to life" has been circulating in my head. I thought it was in reference to "bare life". Naked or nude? I have asked myself. Which is the more appropriate term? And what is the difference? One is born nude but certainly not naked; one is born into a web of relations, to a language, that is, to a world where sense circulates and which *makes* sense (in every sense), however senseless this world may appear. At least, this is how Hannah Arendt understood nativity – born to a language, to a World. Across the distance of their different philosophies, these notions also correspond with Benjamin's condition of "man," at least in one reading of his inherently, incurably enig-matic "Critique of Violence": "existence, that is 'life' is irreducible to the total condition that is 'man'"; and in an even stronger formulation: "man cannot at any price coincide with the mere life in him" (Benjamin, 1996, p. 251). By consequence, naked or bare life, the *bloße Leben* of Benjamin that Agamben often cites, is secondary; it cannot be the original, the first condition. On the contrary, it comes after, is something extracted from life itself and not the result of a violent separation or dispossession of acquired attributes and qualifications. In other words, bare life is the product of an operation and, as such, is not a thing. It is relational, possible only within a structure imposed in/by/through a political relation.

I soon realize that the syntagma's origin is Aristotle, or rather Agamben's reading of Aristotle's *Politics*: "man is born with regard to life but exist[(s] essentially with regard to good life." Aristotle's categorical distinction is in fact the kernel of Agamben's "biopolitical" thesis: the original political relation is the exclusion of existence as bare life. It also allows for a different reading of Benjamin's enigma, one that forces the ambivalence mentioned above in the other direction – that of a moral contempt for the ignominy (Benjamin's term) of a life that would voluntarily choose bare life, clinging on to existence at all cost, to nothing but the bare life (in life). In other words, a contempt for the Italians in their willingness to surrender every political right, even sociality (family, friendship, funerals), to escape from the sickness of the virus. (This same moral contempt may also explain why, many decades ago, Agamben advised Jean-Luc Nancy not have the heart transplant that saved his life.) For confirmation, Agamben again cites Aristotle: "if there is no great difficulty as to the way of life [*kata ton bion*], clearly most men will tolerate much suffering and hold onto life (*zoe*) as if it were a kind of serenity [*euemereia*, beautiful day] and a natural sweetness" (Agamben, 1998, p. 2).

Something, however, remains unaccounted for: the "as if" of Aristotle. As if we could or should read it as casting doubt upon the reality of the "beautiful day" and natural sweetness, or upon what Glenn Gould characterized in Bach's method of composition – its endless detours, delays, and refusal to reach the end – as what matters (in music): the "joyous essence of being".

What if we read Aristotle's "as if" otherwise? Pointing to the founding gesture of the *concept* itself whose own division of the life-world *bios*/*zoe* is founded on the (non-inclusive) exclusion of a remainder: something of life, not bare life but the "beautiful day," which is the remainder of the conceptional division that neither register, neither *bios* (qualified life) nor *zoe* (bare life) can accommodate.

Today, more than ever it seems, we need to return to this unaccounted-for remainder; especially today, at the time of this epidemic, we need to recuperate it from its exile underground, as we – not just the Italians but the whole world – tremble in the face of a globalizing threat to life in each and every one of us.

In Foucault's original construction (invention), the biopolitical opens a path in another possible direction, leading away from drawing any direct or indirect line between the agonizing body of the coronavirus patient in the hospital bed and the death camp ("the nomos of the modern political"). This new paradigm of governmentality takes charge of life, even if only life and nothing but biological life. No matter how reductive a concept of life its bios may be, unlike existence – static, as it were, lifeless – bio is "vital," the terrain of dynamic articulations, the encounter of forces/intensities/sensations. In the original construction, the concept cuts up things in the world differently; its new political invests itself in life, manages living, the biological existence of the living, whose powers it enhances, whose force and capacities it amplifies and augments, whose life span it prolongs (see Michel Serres's celebrations of the biopolitical advances made in the last century: the eradication of diseases, the reduction of poverty and hunger, the extension of life expectancy, etc. across the world). For this reason, the biopolitical is embarrassed in the face of death as evidence or proof of its failure. (Hence one more reason for the embarrassment at the rising number of infections and the death toll. Trump lies about it; the Russians, the Iranians and, at the outbreak, the Chinese try to hide it.)

It is perhaps safe to say that the political response to the pandemic has been biopolitical in Foucault's classical definition of the concept: a practice of governmentality that takes charge of the ensemble of the living, in this case, of the mechanics of life as concerns the health, hygiene, survival, and death of a *population*. ("Flattening the curve" is exemplary in this regard: it is concerned with the survival *rate* of the population and hence with "herd immunity," the spread and incidence of the infection over time, and not with the life of the individual (saving lives)). But it would be an error to deduce from this that the reactive agent itself is the same old biopolitical. In the age of mondialization – when "population" is fluid, constantly de- and re-constituted at different geographic locations by a mobile and migrant capital in search of the lowest cost – governmental practices have long renounced the one form of biopower, namely, the fostering of life, and aggressively maintained instead only the other component, withdrawing from life to the point of death. Rather than a continued extension/expansion of biopolitics, the current emergency measures are reactivations of old forms. The virus forces governments to rediscover the "population" they abandoned long ago; or rather, it itself reconstitutes or recomposes, with great force, the masses of disparate, atomized bodies living in cities, regions, and states into the living body of a collective collectively exposed, infected and infectious, contaminated and contaminating,[4] just as it exposes the impower of the digital, the virtual, the artificial, the gig economy, the forces of immaterialization, derivatives, bitcoin, the financial industry, and the power of life and of the material real (masks, ventilators, protective clothing, medicines; the daily food supply, life-saving medicines, even toilet paper). Just as it exposes the extraordinary and extraordinarily unexploited power of the living *body* of the most downtrodden, the "essential" labor of migrants and minorities; of the truck driver, the janitor, the garbage collector, the bus driver, the mailman, the cashier, the distributor, the grocery clerk, the fireman, the delivery man; of orderlies and caregivers in old-age homes, workers in meat processing plants, seasonal agricultural laborers, and by extension, those hands responsible for milking cows, feeding pigs, gathering eggs, baking breads, picking fruits, and so forth.

If it is not (necessarily/immediately) in the hospital bed, in the intubated body hooked up to a ventilator, that we find bare life today, then where is it? What region of this globalized political is its proper habitat? Has it vanished from the theater of the political? In fact, it is everywhere (different geological planes/plates of the political co-exist, are contiguous, in the same chronological time). It is, for example, the body bobbing in the Mediterranean Sea, clinging onto the side of a packed inflatable; it is the body "kettled" behind barbed-wire fencing off camps on all sides at both edges of Europe; it is caged into the enclave outside Idlib, Syria, and crowded onto a sliver of dry land between two bodies of filthy water on the border between Bangladesh and Myanmar.

The question is, then, how to rescue what necessarily falls in between, exists in the gap between life's nakedness and its full qualification (person, personality, the singularity of its quality), between political life and bare life? How to rescue by way of a concept or concepts the sweetness Aristotle spoke of and rescue it as irreducible to fear (of death), to instinct (of survival), clinging onto life at any cost (which earns Agamben's contempt and Benjamin's characterization as ignoble)? How to rescue that element or dimension – but what is the right word here? Is it not sense? – the *sense* (in every sense of this word) of life, whose "non-existence would be something more terrible" (says Benjamin) than any "attained" condition of man?

The body clinging onto the side of an overcrowded inflatable, the body that makes one last effort to cross the desert, is bare life: standing in a relation, even in it its absolute solitude and abandonment. It is a creation, a product manufactured by the machinery of a political that expelled it precisely from the world into which it was born – in fact, from the World itself; outside the law but held by the law outside the World. On the other hand, what *Aquarius* and the other rescue ships are searching for in the open sea, what the volunteers combing the desert of Texas for refugees hope to save, is a third category of living existence. Deleuze (2001) gave it the simple name: *a* life:

> No one has described better what *a* life is than Charles Dickens. . . . A disreputable man, a rogue, held in contempt by everyone, is found as he lies dying. Suddenly those taking care of him manifest an eagerness, respect, even love, for his slightest sign of life. Everybody bustles about to save him, to the point, where, in the deepest coma, this wicked man senses something soft and sweet penetrating him [Aristotle's "beautiful day?"]. . . . Between his life and his death, there is a moment that is only that of *a* life playing with death. (p. 28)

Even in animals, or rather, in our relation to animals, we distinguish between bare life and *a* life: animals are killed en masse – think of mass fishing – without committing a crime. But when residents along a coastline rush to save a few whales that have beached themselves, pushing and pulling them, watering their skin against the heat of the sun until the next tide comes in, what they respond to in each instance is *a* life, a single and singular life passing through this or that body of a giant animal.

The patient lying on the hospital bed, gasping for air, doctors bustling about him, is a patient-body, a sick-body wherein *a* life is combatting death. "The life of an individual gives way to an impersonal yet singular life that releases a pure event freed from the accidents of internal and external life. . . : 'Homo tantum.'" The life of an individuality (what Benjamin called "qualities" and "attributes") "fades away in favor of a singular life immanent to a man who no longer has a name" (Deleuze, 2001).

This pure event is beyond the reach (re-territorialization) of every economy, calculation, measure, or comparison. It is something the political, biopolitical or not, cannot possibly grasp or touch, even if the medical personages, its agents or actors, respond to it instantaneously, intuitively, without necessarily understanding it. And when the political does touch it, when its relative value – relative to another life, to its utility or the life years it still has left to live – is measured on the scale of a point system of "last resort guidelines," then this pure event of *a* life is instantaneously converted into nothing more than bare life. When the ventilator is removed (or not) to help another patient survive, *both* become nothing more than bare life, more or less deserving to live according to a measured and measurable "merit."

Postscript

Just as I finish drafting this text (without finishing with any of the questions the inventive virus keeps throwing at us, differently every day), Viktor Orbán of Hungary extends by decree the previously declared state of emergency, claiming indefinite powers for his office, indefinitely.

Hungary: is this final accomplishment of "illiberal" democracy a vindication a posteriori of Agamben's much criticized (rather than critiqued) contribution to the question? Did he foresee it, did he predict its coming; that the virus will be turned into a political weapon, and not only by Orbán, and become the pretext for the state of emergency becoming the normal form of government?

Once again, is it not just the form? (Form is relatively stable, but the content varies (Nietzsche). Is it not just the form that is turned into a weapon, in the service not of a biopolitical regime carried to its very limit but, in the case of Hungary, of an archaic, despotic kleptocracy? (Hungary has no experience of democratic forms of government, not even in its most reduced formalistic version now practiced elsewhere/everywhere.) Instead of an exercise in biopower, the new political regime in Hungary stands in a relation of grotesque symmetry with that other regime of illimitation, that of Bolsonaro in Brazil, whose rhetoric incites public "incontinence" – promiscuous consumption, including the consumption by fire of the Amazon forest and its "river in the sky" that brings the rains to Africa.

What future path the globalized world will breach for itself one cannot know. Whether it will try (in vain) to return the world to what it was just a few months ago (although it seems like a lifetime); or worse, make the economy "roar" like a spruced-up car engine; or, on the contrary, it will learn the lesson this virus may teach us regarding the other existential crisis, which will not go away, even if we have almost lost sight of it in the midst of this immediate emergency? The lesson is that de-carbonization is possible. The skies over Mumbai are blue again, the sea around Venice has been taken over by wildlife. Whether this lesson – mercilessly delivered by nothing more than a few strings of molecules, dormant, waiting for a life to come along to live – will be learnt, one cannot say. All that can be said is that what the "after" might be is yet to be determined.

Now this "viral" lesson, harsh and cruel as it may be, curiously resembles the divine justice of Benjamin. It does not spill blood, and it kills without leaving a trace of the act – in the interest of life, without a trace: after the epidemic has passed and the generation responsible – if only through complicity – for the geocide on course will have been decimated, there will be no memory of the act. In the interest of life: perhaps it is a chance, perhaps the only chance, for another future for, made by, another (the "Greta") generation.

Notes

1 I am writing this at the beginning of April, only a few short weeks after Agamben's first intervention, during which period the virus has escaped definitions, evaded defensive measures, outpaced projections, predictions, prognoses. This viral inventiveness, however, is only one reason why I will not engage Agamben regarding the nature of the virus nor predicate on it the discussion here.
2 According to the latest, in all likelihood, "conspiracy theory," it escaped from the P4 high-security bio-lab of Wuhan and from the control of the scientists or lab technicians who created it, or at least sought precisely to take charge of it, learn how to master it, and manipulate its code. This paranoid fantasy speaks to the dominant relation, even if it overestimates the power of science over life.
3 In this partial and selective destruction, the virus resembles the neutron bomb designed to kill only the living while leaving (dead) infrastructure untouched. The virus, on the other hand, attacks the World, the living space of making (creating) sense, where sense circulates and is exchanged; it empties cities, theaters and the cinema; turns to deserts public spaces of gathering, of protestation, and mourning and celebration, where one makes an appearance, becomes visible – all the while leaving/passing through other living forms (bats, pangolins) without leaving a trace.
4 This curious forgetting of population would need to be reflected on at length. Here I can only defer to Foucault's argument in 2008 (*The Birth of Biopolitics*) that in certain forms of neoliberalism economy detaches itself from society to enter into a reciprocal, symbiotic relation with the political: the political authorizes economic operations which in turn legitimize the political. The excluded third, the social (health, welfare, housing, etc.), enters the ledger of negative expenditures.

References

Agamben, G. (1998). *Homo sacer: Sovereign power and bare life*. Stanford University Press.
Agamben, G. (2005). *State of exception* (K. Attel, Trans.). University of Chicago Press.
Agamben, G. (2020a). Clarifications. *European Journal of Psychoanalysis*. www.journal-psy-choanalysis.eu/coronavirus-and-philosophers/

Agamben, G. (2020b, March 24). L'épidémie montre clairement que l'état d'exception est devenu la condition normale [The epidemic clearly demonstrations that the state of exception has become the normal condition]. *Le Monde.* www.lemonde.fr/idees/article/2020/03/24/giorgio-agamben-l-epidemie-montre-clairement-que-l-etat-d-exception-est-devenu-la-condition-normale_6034245_3232.html

Agamben, G. (2020c, February 26). L'invenzione di un'epidemia [The invention of an epidemic]. *Quodlibet.* www.quodlibet.it/giorgio-agamben-l-invenzione-di-un-epidemia [European Journal of Psychoanalysis. www.journal-psychoanalysis.eu/coronavirus-and-philosophers/]

Arendt, H. (1958). *The human condition.* University of Chicago Press.

Benjamin, W. (1996). Critique of violence. In *Selected writings* (Vol. 1). Harvard University Press.

Deleuze, G. (2001). Immanence: A life. In A. Boyman (Trans.), *Pure immanence: Essays on a life.* Zone Books.

Foucault, M. (1990). Right of death and power over life. In R. Hurley (Trans.), *The history of sexuality* (Vol. 1). Vintage Books. (Original work published 1976)

Foucault, M. (2008). *The birth of the biopolitics: Lectures at the Collège de France, 1978–1979* (G. Burchell, Trans.). Palgrave Macmillan.

11 A much too human virus

Jean-Luc Nancy
April 13, 2020

As has often been said, Europe has been exporting its wars since 1945. Having fallen apart, it was unable to do anything but spread its disunion through its old colonies, and along the lines of its alliances and competing interests with the new power poles of the world. Between these poles, Europe was only a memory, while still pretending to have a future.

And now, Europe is importing. Not only merchandise, as it has long done, but first and foremost populations – something that is not new either but that is becoming urgent, even overwhelming – at a pace set by the conflicts it exports and by environmental problems (which also originated in Europe). Today, Europe is importing a viral epidemic.

What does this mean? It is not simply a question of the spread, which has its vectors and trajectories. Europe is not the center of the world – far from it – but it persists in playing its long-standing role as a model or an example. Elsewhere, there may be very strong attractions and impressive opportunities. Some are traditional, perhaps old-fashioned, like in North America; others are newer, in Asia and Africa (with South America being a special case, where many European features are combined with other particularities). But Europe seemed, or believed itself to be, more or less desirable, at least as a refuge.

The old theatre of the exemplary – justice, science, democracy, beauty and well-being – attracts desires, even if these desires attach themselves to worn out or even outmoded objects. Thus, Europe stays open to visitors although it is not welcoming for those who cannot pay for such desires. It is not surprising, then, that a virus enters the picture.

Nor is it surprising that in Europe this virus creates greater confusion than in the place of its origin. Indeed, China had already established order with regard to markets as well as diseases. Europe, on the other hand, was in a state of relative disorder: between nations and between aspirations. This led to some indecision, agitation and difficult adaptation. By contrast, the United States immediately fell back on its grandiose isolationism and its unhesitating ability to decide. Europe has always been trying to find itself – and the world, which it kept discovering, exploring and exploiting – after which still not knowing where it stood.

Just when the first epicenter of the pandemic seemed to have been brought under control, and many countries not yet affected closed their doors to Europeans and to the Chinese, Europe became the epicenter of the pandemic. It was there that we saw the accumulated effects of travel to China (business, leisure, studies), of visitors from China and elsewhere (business, leisure, studies), of its own general uncertainties and, finally, of its internal dissention.

It would be tempting to summarize the situation like this: in Europe it is "Run for your life" and elsewhere it is "Show me what you're made of, virus!" Or like this: in Europe, the dillydallying, the skepticism and the hardheadedness are more prevalent than in many other places. This is our "reasoning reason" legacy, libertine and libertarian; in other words, the legacy we, old Europeans, considered the very life of the mind.

This is why the inevitable reiteration of the expression "exceptional measures" resuscitates the ghost of Carl Schmitt, through a kind of hasty parallel. Thus, the virus spreads the discourses of ostentatious defiance. Showing that you are not fooled is more important than avoiding the contagion – which amounts to being doubly fooled – and perhaps by poorly repressed anxiety, or by a childish feeling of omnipotence or daring.

Everyone (me included) has a comment to make, be it doubtful or attempting an interpretation. Philosophy, psychoanalysis and politology of the virus all have a message to bring.

(Let us accept the view presented by Michel Deguy, in his poem *Coronation*, on the website of the journal *Po&sie*.[1])

Everyone wants to discuss and argue, since we are long used to dealing with difficulties, ignorance and undecidedness. At the global level, what dominates, it seems to me, are confidence, mastery and decision. At least, this is the image that seems to emerge, or to take shape in the collective imagination.

The coronavirus pandemic is, on every level, a product of globalization. It highlights the latter's characteristics and tendencies. It is an active, combative and effective free-trade agent. It takes part in the wider process through which a culture becomes undone, to be replaced by something which is less a culture and more a system of forces indistinguishably technical, economic, authoritarian and sometimes psychological or physical (if we think of oil or the atom). Of course, this process brings into question the economic development model, so that the French president feels obliged to report on it. It is quite possible that we shall have to change our algorithms – but there is no proof that this will serve to usher in a new era.

Indeed, eradicating a virus is not enough. If technical and political mastery proves to be like its outcome, it will only turn the world into a field of forces tensed and pitted against each other, henceforth stripped of any of the civilizing elements that came into play previously. The contagious brutality of the virus spreads as administrative brutality. We are already dealing with the need to select those eligible for treatment. (And this is not counting the inevitable economic and social injustices.) This is not some underhanded plot devised by an unknown sinister conspirator, nor is it the result of abuses on the part of nations. The only thing at work is the general law of interconnections, whose mastery is the aim of techno-economic powers.

In the past, pandemics could be considered divine punishment, just as illness in general was seen for a very long time as external to the social body. Today, most illnesses are endogenous, caused by our living conditions, the quality of our food and the toxicity of our environment. What used to be divine has become human – too human, as Nietzsche says. For a long time, modernity could be defined according to Pascal's formula, "Man infinitely surpasses man". But if he surpasses himself "too much", that is, without rising to the Pascalian divine – then he does not surpass himself at all. Instead, he becomes mired in a humanity overwhelmed by the events and situations it has produced.

Indeed, the virus confirms the absence of the divine, since we know its biological nature. We are even discovering how much more complex and harder to define living beings are, than we had previously described them to be. We are also discovering to what extent the exercise of political power – that of a people, that of a so-called community, like the "European" community or a military dictatorship – is another form of complexity, once again harder to define than we might have thought. We understand better now how inadequate the term "biopolitics" is in these conditions. Life and politics challenge us together. Our scientific knowledge tells us that we are dependent only on our own technical power, but there is no pure technicity because the knowledge itself includes uncertainties (one only has to read the published studies). Because technical power is not unequivocal, how much less unequivocal must a political power be, while supposedly guided by objective data, and expected to respond to legitimate expectations?

Of course, decisions must nevertheless be based on presumed objectivity. If this objectivity dictates "confinement" or "distancing", how far should authorities go to enforce them? And of course, inversely, at what point can we speak of the vested interests of a government that wants – for example – to preserve the Olympic Games from which it expects to profit, as do many businesses and sports managers in whose behalf the government is acting as well? Or the interests of a government which takes this opportunity to rekindle nationalist feelings?

The viral magnifying glass enlarges the characteristics of our contradictions and of our limitations. It is a reality principle that collides with the pleasure principle. Death is its companion. Death that we exported with wars, famines and devastation, that we thought we confined to a few other viruses and to cancers (now in quasi-viral expansion), now waits for us around the corner. What do you know! We are humans, two-legged, without feathers and gifted with language, but certainly neither superhuman nor transhuman. Too human? Or are we to understand that there can be no such thing as "too" human, and that it is precisely this which surpasses us infinitely?

Note

1 See https://po-et-sie.fr/chroniques/coronation/

12 The return of Antigone

Burial rites in pandemic times

Néstor Braunstein
May 25, 2020

A notable essay by my friend Asunción Álvarez (2020) sparked these reflections on burial rites and their imposed modifications due to the present circumstances, which can only be defined as a "state of exception." This name risks incurring in non-sense or an oxymoron, since the claim is that we must adapt to a "new normal," the interruption of a previous legal order regarding basic rights, such as the freedom of assembly, commerce, travel within the city and beyond its borders, and so forth. The Covid-19 pandemic altered an otherwise "normal" condition, and a "state of exception" has been established, like it or not.[1]

For many, myself included, the state of emergency implies a dictatorial infringement of basic civil liberties, which large segments of the population justify and accept, albeit resignedly, due to the supposed belief that these measures prevent contagion and fatalities. The long history of a paternalistic logic of biopower is at work here: "It is for your own good that we order you to do it!" In the new world order that is outlined before our eyes, Big Brother restricts privacy, making the latter an increasingly archaic term. Health is equivalent to wealth in the war for planetary economic power, which states administer and regulate.

The rites and norms that regulate certain behaviors regarding the bodies of the dead can be counted among the new conditions that the state enforces. Under habitual, "normal" conditions in "democratic" societies, the people closest to the deceased were allowed to decide, even before death, on the funeral rites to be followed. Countries and cities were governed by specific rules and procedures regulating the steps to take. We will not dwell on this point; there is a generalized consensus that this is as it should be. A cultural universal, we might say, obvious and widely known, is embedded in the set of citizens' legitimate and legal freedoms.

This central issue is rigorously detailed in the text by A. Álvarez. I congratulated the author upon reading it and noted that its implications brought us back to the time of Antigone, Creon and Polynices, as we know them from multiple sources, especially Sophocles's tragedy. Although the present circumstances also brought to mind my previous work on this subject presented at a colloquium on funerary art in Mexico, I will not limit myself to those earlier reflections here.[2] I wish to go further by examining, from the perspective of the present, one of the main points of that work: the condition of those who live "between two deaths," according to an invaluable contribution by the Marquis de Sade (2015 [1797]) at the end of the 18th century and later taken up by Jacques Lacan in his seminar of May and June in 1960 (1992). A month ago, G. Agamben wrote about the legal restrictions imposed due to the pandemic, reflecting on the limits we would not tolerate were they transgressed in the name of public health safety. The Italian philosopher focused on three characteristics of the supposed "new normality." I will translate only the first one:

> The first point, perhaps the most serious, concerns the bodies of the deceased persons. How can we have accepted, for the sake of a *risk* impossible to specify, that persons we love and human beings in general, should not only die alone – something that had never occurred in history from Antigone until now – but their corpse be incinerated without any burial rites?
>
> (Agamben, 2020a)

Antigone had returned. I re-read my text of some 40 years ago where, based on Lacan's works, I wrote about burial rites and the figure of Antigone. I found it reasonable enough to re-think Agamben's question but considered a re-appraisal necessary because of important essays published in the intervening years. Those texts, which I will discuss shortly, as well as Álvarez's article, offer an opportunity to once again return to the beautiful and uncanny figure of Antigone. It allows us to reflect on the consequences of the present regulation of burial rites that prescribe what is allowed and not allowed, and how past norms are being modified under the pretext of public health. Antigone can still teach us a great deal with her own example: a destiny, chosen in defiance of the despotic tyrant claiming to act on behalf of the salvation (health) of the city.

What can and should be done with the bodies of the dead in pandemic times? Are these bodies dangerous due to the risk of contagion? How much time should transpire between death and the burial or cremation of the bodily remains? What must be done with their clothing and other personal objects that could be contaminated? What of the wakes, masses, lay and religious ceremonies, the gatherings of mourners and friends? Few, if any, of these questions have a clear answer in 2020.

Due to the pandemic and fear of infection, the time allowed for a deceased body to be present before it reaches its destination has accelerated: it must be disposed of quickly and as soon as possible. New cemeteries must be built quickly. The gravediggers cannot keep up. There are not enough coffins and the dead are often buried in cardboard boxes or plastic bags, such as those thrown into the garbage bins found in the corners of large cities. Latin America, with Brazil and Ecuador as the most extreme and impoverished, is at the forefront of this degradation of life even in death. The profanation of the corpse is common and points to an anti-erotic, thanatotic force, especially if we agree with

G. Bataille (1986 [1957]): "Erotism is the affirmation of life, even in death" (p. 83). We can invert the formula in light of the present cancellation of burial rites: "Anti-erotism is the condemnation of death in the name of life."

We all know there is historical variability in the norms and customs of different sectors of societies, cultures, and religions regarding their more or less specific rituals. We also know that for some time now, in the West at least, death has lost its status as a decisive event. The classic, essential work on this topic is by Philippe Ariès (1981), while the banalization of death is Agamben's central topic in *Homo Sacer* (1998). Many authors, such as Jean Allouch (2001), refer to the present time, whether to lament it or not, as "dry death": the reduction of the time and external signs of mourning, the generalized desiccation of the flood of tears, the cancellation of hired mourners (*lloronas*), or a widow's self-cremation in certain cultures. In many parts of the postmodern world, the external signs of mourning required in the past have become shameful, as if they were an invitation to explain or speak about why they are carried out and in that way place the deceased at the forefront of any dialogue with the other.

Now is not the time to speculate on the economic, social, political, and ecological reasons for these changes. These appear to be intimately linked to the secularization of nation states, the acceleration of time corresponding to modern technologies that run at the speed of light, and life expectancy statistically related to advances in the medical treatment of acute and chronic illnesses. The latter make death an expected event due to an aging population, weakened by the span of time and physical decay. The old are now the vulnerable ones, those who can be "disposed of" more rapidly when decisions are made regarding the distribution of the scarce healthcare resources available, the result of cuts justified by neoliberal policies dedicated to more "productive" ends.

Old age is costly when considering the economic and human resources dedicated to its needs. "Retirement homes" (in many cases a euphemism for a "depository") are real estate, a superfluous expenditure given that its residents have nothing to contribute. With Swiftian humor ("A Modest Proposal for Preventing the Children of Poor People from Being a Burthen to their Parents, or the Country, and for Making them Beneficial to the Publick," 1729), problems could be resolved with a "final solution," Eichmann style. British Prime Minister Boris Johnson was not far off from such a proposal when he claimed it would resolve the issue of caring for useless old people and would contribute to herd immunity, which the active part of the population could reach via geronticide. In Mexico, the expression used is *desviejadero*.[3]

Death in the 21st century is not what it used to be. It has become naturalized and thus lost its supernatural aspect. There is no need for statistics to know how many people believe or not in eternal life, heaven, purgatory, paradise, and the promises, performative and impossible to invalidate, regarding the resurrection of bodies (who can declare the promise was not kept?). The mandate of a virtuous life needed to secure or achieve an otherworldly reward is now put aside in favor of the order to enjoy early and as much as possible. What seems to prevail now is the rather vulgar saying: "the living to enjoy, the dead to the hole" (*el vivo al gozo y el muerto al pozo*). That hole is no longer the site of pilgrimages, care, and floral ornaments. Cemeteries are losing the halo of being saintly ground. The mandate to forget is preferred to the Hebrew *zachor* as well to the Passion in Christian mass. In present day anti-erotics one must turn the page as soon as possible. It's time to move on!

The facts are here with us and underscored in these times of exception, be it because of the need to avoid crowds around the deceased due to the potential danger of the corpse or because the bereaved cannot travel in this era of globalization, when practically everyone has family and friends abroad or at a great distance from the place of origin (the means of transport are impossible to find or one risks being quarantined when arriving or departing). Everything conspires to modify burial rites, those sublime *Totenfeier* of Mahler's Second Symphony or the many versions of the Requiem Mass, including the death and resurrection of Jesus Christ every Easter (Reik, 1953). In 2020 the Christian liturgy was interrupted for the first time since the Middle Ages with the Vatican's consent, although not without local resistance. It was one of the many although not the least important ways by which the "state of exception" was manifested.

At best, the commemoration of the dead is postponed until after the quarantine period, when sports events can also be rescheduled. Meanwhile, funerals can only be attended by ten people and transmitted by social media for those not present. The coffins must be closed. The contact with the deceased's body or clothing is prohibited, as are thanatoesthetics and lustral washes, the cleansing of the dead. In the United States, President Trump ordered the flag be flown at half-mast when the country reached 100,000 dead, and in Spain, President Pedro Sánchez decreed ten days of national mourning. These are collective commemorations that blur the restrictions placed on the bereaved. Thousands, instead of each one, with their anonymous and embarrassing dead. Some Jewish and Muslim religious leaders decided against revealing the time and place of religious ceremonies to limit the influx of worshippers. In various parts of Mexico, there have been attacks on the vehicles that transport the health professionals who care for the sick, and even on hearses.

One could say that this is the context for the induced and premeditated paranoia of a global experiment conducted on behalf of "biosecurity," according to the definition Agamben (2020b) provides in a recently published text. Under penalty of death, the world's population is impelled toward a "voluntary servitude," as La Boétie (2016 [1576]) once noted. The control of bodies and their movements, contacts, the distances between them, and so forth looms on the horizon thanks to sensors that transmit the variables through apps installed in devices connected to the internet. In China and South Korea, those devices are already in general use and are credited with being responsible for the successful control of the pandemic. The UK appears to be the next client in line for this voluntary servitude. It is not science fiction. The future is here. One must protect oneself from this virus and if not this one, the next. There is no better protection against terror than the creation of an even greater one. Gatherings of people, especially in great numbers, are dangerous; it is best for each one to be isolated, using technological devices. The body of the *socius* contaminates, the emblematic *ágora* is at risk: Hyde Park, the liberal institution and space of a legendary London, becomes Hidden Park.[4]

Each change and restriction the *polis* imposes regarding burial rites recalls and commemorates the emblematic tragedy of Antigone that Sophocles (ca. 440 BCE) dramatized in exemplary manner. It is one of the West's great myths, adapted to all literary and artistic genres in innumerable versions, as George Steiner (1994) noted. These versions continue to grow. It is difficult to find the name of any well-known thinker who has not concerned herself or himself with Antigone, fruit of the incestuous love between Oedipus and Jocasta, who confronts her maternal uncle, the tyrant Creon, King of Thebes, demanding burial rites for her brother Polynices, condemned to die without them. Surprisingly missing from that list of thinkers is Sigmund Freud, whose keen knowledge of the theater and Greek myths made the history and destiny of Oedipus, Antigone's father, a central focus of his theory of the psyche. The young maiden does not appear in the index of names in Freud's *Collected Works*, even though in later years Freud privately identifies himself with the tragic hero and calls his beloved daughter, Anna Freud ("a possession"), his Antigone.[5]

As if signaling Freud's omission, his disciple or epigone Jacques Lacan dedicated various classes to Antigone in his 1960 seminar on the ethics of psychoanalysis. These classes that show a profound and unfathomable erudition have been the object of serious and detailed readings by those who follow Lacan's teachings. We are no exception. Agamben (2020a) turns to the young heroine as the prototype of the resistance of family to the law of the city, embodied by the despot that rules its destiny. Creon decrees the state of exception, condemning Polynices to die without sepulture as the enemy of the *polis* of Thebes, and is thrown to the dogs and birds of prey. Antigone evokes another law that differs from the tyrant's and that for her is superior: a law that is chthonic (of the earth), of the mother, in confrontation with a celestial, phallocratic power. In our 1980 conference we indicated seven points of conflict that could be applied to the present situation emerging from the unexpected but anticipated outbreak of a virus against which there are no antidotes for now and that casts its pestilence over all nation states. Those seven points are the following:

1   The central relation of Antigone against Creon, which Hegel emphasizes as the opposition between the rights of the family and those of the state.
2   The relation between Antigone and Polynices, her brother, which is Sophocles's focus.
3   The antagonic (Antigonic?) relation between masculine and feminine, underlined in the discussion between Creon and Haemon, the former's son and Antigone's betrothed. The tyrant confronts his son thus: "It is very clear that you have become the ally of a woman."
4   The conflict between Antigone the rebel and her sister Ismene: opposing sides between feminine rebellion and submission to masculine domination.

5   Antigone's relation to Jocasta's maternal desire. Jocasta, Polynices' mother, cannot accept the infamy that a child born of her entrails should not have proper sepulture.
6   The acceptance of *até*, Antigone's tragic destiny, which entails accepting oneself a criminal without guilt or remorse and for this reason facing the atrocious punishment of descending to her own sepulture while still alive.
7   The defiance of what is most terrible, uncanny, *Unheimliche* (Freud, 1919); the suffocation Antigone suffers when her executioners bury her alive.

Our text, still current in 2020, unpacked those seven conflicts. In his seminar (1992), Lacan emphasized what is our interest now: the condition of the dead without sepulture. They remain between two deaths. Antigone is their paradigm: the first death is natural, an interruption of the vital processes, the specular image and the word. The second death is annihilating and irrevocable, eliminating the symbolic and imaginary rests as well as the sepulture of a former living being who had a proper name, spoken as "I," and was considered a member of society. Power, in the name of the public good, commands the erasure of memory. It is the too frequent situation of the "disappeared," which we do not know if they are living or dead, where and when to find them or no longer look for them; those without sepulture, which in stories of zombies wander among the living demanding remembrance and recognition.

They are also the "archived" elderly who now die in "residences," forgotten by all, considered un-privileged carriers of pestilence, the most vulnerable, putrid carrion whose stench must disappear immediately, without leaving any remains able to contaminate those who enter into contact with what was formerly a body and is now mere flesh. The flesh of a human being becomes body when it enters language, gives it a name, and attaches it to a specular image that constitutes its "identity." In Guayaquil, Ecuador, for example, many are not placed in coffins but rather are carried away in cardboard boxes, thrown in common graves, pits, and holes in the ground that become signifiers of the annihilating will of the Other.

The pandemic makes holes in the earth for the dead without names; they remain in those barren spaces, comparable to point zero at Hiroshima or Nagasaki, the Twin Towers, Chernobyl, Fukushima, or the plastic islands that contaminate oceans. The planet is filling up with ominous grounds that signal a topology and toponomy where persons remain "between two deaths," mute witnesses of a humanity fading in oblivion. The state claims the authority to consider the body of the deceased, the corpse, a "thing" and deny it the status of "person," against established legislation and jurisprudence (Toureil-Divina, 2015). The dead cannot demand their rights, but those who survive them can. It is not a trivial question: we will all be corpses in an unpredictable but not distant future and, as such, it is in defense of liberty that we argue for the right to decide over the destiny of our own remains. The respect for the body is not over when animate life ends; it is an attribute of personal dignity. For this reason, in the articles by Agamben and Álvarez we've discussed, there is an emphasis on the elimination of rituals, the inalienable rights of she or he who had a place in a genealogy, were inscribed in language and should not be treated as a piece of furniture. Among these rights is of course the personal choice to eliminate burial rites: cremation or the scattering of ashes on earth or water, or even other possibilities, such as embalming, cryopreservation, or perhaps at the limits of science fiction, the sending off to outer space or keeping death in suspense, as in Edgar Allen Poe's *Strange Case of M. Valdemar* (1844).

From the perspective of Lacanian psychoanalysis, one must take into account the desire to express a "last wish," notarized or not. Here one can clearly see that the deceased is desiring, although not *jouissante* (*gozante*) because there is only jouissance in life and in the movement of the drives, activated by corporal sources.[6] The corpse does not *jouit* (*goza*) but is the object of the desire of the Other, as well as those others (widows or widowers, sons or daughters of first and second marriages) who can agree or not regarding the destination of the body: the disposition of the place and arrangement of the burial rites, the task of undertakers, the sale of lots and pantheons in specific locations throughout the city, even the sepulture of pets (see E. Waugh, *The Loved One* [1948]). All these belong to the jouissance of the Other, including the power of the state, the power of present-day Creons to *jouir* the bodies of the Labdacids, extinguished because they had no offspring.

This is why burial rites are needed: they make death a social event and not an individual avatar. The corpse can no longer participate in the social link that speech establishes but can be a link for the social (*lien social*). The rite brings together the survivors that evoke memory, the fame or infamy of the deceased. The burial rite establishes, historicizes, and questions the bereaved's memory and those who will undertake their singular grieving process by incorporating and making their own the symbolic and imaginary traces of the deceased. Mozart is the epitome of this destiny, but Lacan also mentions other examples when he writes: "No doubt a corpse is a signifier, but Moses' tomb is as empty for Freud as Christ's was for Hegel" (*Écrits*, 2006, p. 693). Mozart is irrevocably lost for the Viennese. The Holy Sepulcher justified centuries-old wars whose echoes linger to this day.

In Sophocles's *Oedipus at Colonus*, Oedipus and Creon dispute the proper place for Oedipus's own sepulture. In that confrontation, Theseus, King of Athens, mediates by affirming that good luck and blessedness, as well as the loving affection of the Athenians, will bring fortune to the citizens of the nation that would welcome Oedipus's remains. Creon had wanted to seize the body of the old and blind Oedipus by force and take it to the city where the latter had been king (see *Oedipus Rex*). Although the play is the last of Sophocles's known works, the action that unfolds in *Oedipus at Colonus* is prior to the tragic events that occur in *Antigone*. For this reason, in *Oedipus at Colonus*, Oedipus's four children (Eteocles, Polynices, Antigone, and Ismene) are the ones who argue about the rites and site where their father's remains should lie. The West wavers, even today, in the midst of a pandemic, between the graveyard and the dissemination of ashes after an industrial cremation. Where should lifeless bodies be placed?

In the space "between two deaths," Antigone suffers misfortunes (*atê*) in the place the tyrant reserves for her brother. Rebelling against the decree of the king who represents the *polis*, Antigone secures her brother a sepulcher. By claiming *autonomy*, she immortalizes her crime and denounces political power. Her destiny is comparable to those "dead without a sepulcher": the corpses of Argentines cast to sea from airplanes, Don Juan thrown to Hell, Captain Ahab drowned by Leviathan's fury (Moby Dick) and falling from his boat into the storm at sea, Job the prophet – all those who dare rebel against the supreme authority, much like Leonard Bernstein in his Third Symphony, *Kaddish*. Let us recall that Kaddish, the traditional Jewish prayer for the dead, is not a hymn for their remembrance but a prayer to extol God.

Our remarks could well end on this point, but a final clarification is in order to avoid confusion and abusive over-simplifications regarding the issue, limiting the discussion to a question of how to dispose of bodily remains in name of the needs of communities, with the pretext of guarding public health. The question is more complex and goes beyond the conflict between Antigone and Creon. It must be approached from a triple perspective: public health, law, and politics:

1   From the *juridical point of view*, which was emphasized here, there is no doubt. The rights of the survivors and those of the deceased must be respected. The latter are neither things nor disposable remains.
2   From the *perspective of public health*, one cannot underestimate the malevolent power of the virus, regardless of its point of origin. Encouraging the general population to protect itself and maintain proper hygiene is wholly justified. Too many barbarities have been committed by certain officials (especially the presidents of the United States and Brazil) to propose the figure of Antigone as a model of civil disobedience toward political authority. It is clear that the measures taken by more qualified, prudent, and scientifically informed governments are showing the best results where everyone is informed of the risks of ending those measures too soon and thus producing a new outbreak. A well-informed but not terrorized population supports those governments, and that is encouraging.
3   What is alarming is the *juridical-political level*, the focus of the Agamben articles already noted. These are wholly valid even if they do not lead to clear guidelines as to what should be done. What Agamben's articles question was already evident at the beginning of 2020 and are not the effect of the virus. Civil liberties, the weakening of imperfect democracies that still respected the electoral and parliamentary process, the growing intrusiveness of technological and social media, the manipulation of social demands, the re-allocation of resources for healthcare and education toward ecocidal and defense budgets – all this and much more was already present and created anxious discontent in progressive sectors (or more appropriately, on

the left) at the beginning of this now ominous 2020. The time has not yet arrived to yearn for a too recent past in terms of what the future may promise. Rather, we would venture to say that everything that went wrong before will be worse in the future, and no one knows where to look for hope. At the beginning of the year we ourselves did not know what political project or program to support. The pandemic did not create a new situation; it worsened what already existed. The left is between a rock and a hard place. The technology we all use fulfills its pharmacological function: it is both cure and poison. The fascists are conscious of their eventual adversaries' general disorientation. They manipulate and extort with the "face-mask" of public health safety: either surrender civil liberties to the ruling power or choose disease and death; your money or your life!

Translated from the Spanish
by Silvia N. Rosman

Notes

1 See Walter Benjamin (1968 [1942]) and G. Agamben (1999).
2 See N. Braunstein (1981).
3 This term refers to the greater mortality rate of older persons, especially at certain times of the year (Trans).
4 See www.cityofvancouver.us/parksrec/page/hidden-park, as the effect of Covid-19.
5 In a letter to Arnold Zweig on February 25, 1934, Freud notes: "But you must realize that much as I resisted it, destiny has compensated me with the possession of a daughter that, in tragic circumstances, would not be far removed from Antigone."
6 In keeping with the untranslatability of certain Lacanian concepts into English, they remain in the original French here. See Braunstein (2020) for a full discussion of this topic (Trans.).

References

Agamben, G. (1998). *Homo sacer: Sovereign power and bare life* (D. Heller-Rozen, Trans.). Stanford University Press.

Agamben, G. (1999). *Remnants of Auschwitz: The witness and the archive* (D. Heller-Rozen, Trans.). Zone Books.

Agamben, G. (2020a, April 20). Une question [A question]. *Lundi Matin, 239.* https://lundi.am/Une-question

Agamben, G. (2020b, May 24). Biosécurité et politique [Biosecurity and politics]. *Lundi Matin, 243.* https://lundi.am/999-Biosecurite-et-politique

Allouch, J. (2001). *Érotique du deuil au les temps de la mort sèche* [*Erotics of mourning in the time of dry death*] (2nd ed.). EPEL.

Álvarez, A. (2020, May 5). Morir y hacer duelo en tiempos de pandemia [To die and mourn in pandemic times]. *El seminario (Mexico).* https://elsemanario.com/opinion/morir-y-hacer-el-duelo-en-tiempos-de-pandemia-asuncion-alvarez/

Ariès, P. (1981). *The hour of our death* (H. Weaver, Trans.). Oxford University Press.

Bataille, G. (1986). *Erotism: Death and sensuality* (M. Dalwood, Trans.). City Lights Books. (Original work published 1957)

Benjamin, W. (1968). Theses on the philosophy of history. In *Illuminations*. Harcourt Brace. (Original work published 1942)

Braunstein, N. (1981). Un diván para Antígona [A divan for Antigone]. In A. Aparicio, N. Braunstein, & N. Saal (Eds.), *A medio siglo del malestar en la cultura de Sigmund Freud* (pp. 169–190). Siglo XXI.

Braunstein, N. (2020). *Jouissance: A Lacanian concept* (S. Rosman, Trans.). SUNY Press.

Freud, S. (1919). *The uncanny*. Vintage Press.

Lacan, J. (1992). *The seminar of Jacques Lacan, book VII: The ethics of psychoanalysis* (D. Porter, Trans.). Norton.

Lacan, J. (2006). *Écrits* (B. Fink, Trans.). Norton.

Marquis de Sade. (2015). *Juliette ou les prospérités du vice* [*Juliette or vice amply rewarded*]. Editions Humanis. (Original work published 1797)

Reik, T. (1953). *The haunting melody: Psychoanalytic experiences in life and music*. Farrar, Straus and Young.

Steiner, G. (1994). *Antigones*. Yale University Press.

Toureil-Divina, M. (2015). Le droit du défunt [The right of the deceased]. *Communications*, *97*(2), 29–48.

Part II
Philosophers act

13 One health and one home

On the biopolitics of Covid-19

Miguel Vatter
March 31, 2020

The Covid-19 pandemic has rather spectacularly confirmed the relevance of the philosophical paradigm known as biopolitics. Not only are we specimens of a biological species who also happen to organize our lives together through politics, but this pandemic has made it crystal clear how much our politics (and economics) are dependent on our capacity to "govern" or "manage" our species life in relation to non-human life as such.

However, we still do not know how the human response to the coronavirus outbreak will re-articulate the connection between our species life and our political life. To date, the pandemic joins two novel elements that stand in need of further critical and biopolitical thought. The first element is the fact that the coronavirus "jumped" between distinct species. This possibility of a species jump that characterizes viral outbreaks with pandemic potential has led public health experts to speak of a "One Health" model. As defined by the Food and Agriculture Organization, "One Health is an integrated approach for preventing and mitigating health threats at the Animal-Human-Plant-Environment interfaces with the objective of achieving public health, food and nutrition security, sustainable ecosystems and fair trade facilitation" (One Health, n.d.). Thus, the phenomenon of a virus that jumps across species not only confirms the belief (already held by Darwin and Nietzsche) that distinct species do not exist as such but are epiphenomena of a continuum of life in constant becoming (Lemm, 2020). The pandemic also indicates that the species jump has its own biopolitical mirror image in questioning traditional immunitary devices like national boundaries and unequal distribution of wealth. As Judith Butler (2020) and Slavoj Žižek (2020) hurriedly pointed out, the virus is uncannily egalitarian. This fact suggests that nationalist and capitalist conceptualizations of the "Animal-Human-Plant-Environment interfaces" will need to be drastically revised in view of achieving One Health on a planetary scale. But now this expression needs to be read as follows: our conception of health needs to be reoriented by the Oneness of life which performatively denies the naturalized hierarchies and speciesism underpinning social pathologies like classism, racism and sexism.

The second novel element is that the rest of the world followed China in adopting the lockdown of their citizens in their homes as the biopolitical policy

of choice to combat the epidemic. What is the significance of this topologi-
cal choice for our biopolitical response? Philosophers of biopolitics have given
varied answers to this question: some, like Giorgio Agamben (2020a, 2020b),
understand the lockdown as a repetition of the sovereign prerogative to "ban"
certain individuals considered to pose a high risk for the "security" of society.
Others, like Sergio Benvenuto (2020), see the lockdown as accelerating a trend
in advanced capitalist societies towards recovering the ancient Greek idea of
home as "hearth" (Gr. *Hestia*): the original space for the reproduction of life
where the instruments for this reproduction are under our "dominion". As
Carl Schmitt (2014) pointed out decades ago, "the house remains the nucleus
and center of terrestrial life, together with its concrete orders: house and property, matrimony, family and inheritance . . . The fundamental institution of
law, *dominium* or property, receives its name from *domus*" (Section V, para. 1).

However, I think that the shock of Covid-19 has done more than shatter a
Panglossian belief that we lived in the best of all possible worlds, just as it has
done more than reiterate Candide's conclusion that the best path in life is simply
to "tend one's garden" and sell the modest products of one's work at home. Just
like the viral species jump highlights the emergence of One Health, so too this
globalized and highly mediatized – thanks to internet technology – lockdown
has led many more to the renewed conviction that we can no longer continue
to "progress" in the way we have done so far. The direct link between a human
species in lockdown and skies free of pollution, old waterways teeming again
with life and so forth has reinforced the most ancient awareness that nature is
the *One Home for humanity*. This explains the sentiment expressed by commen-
tators like George Monbiot (2020), who believes this pandemic "could be the
moment when we begin to see ourselves, once more, as governed by biology
and physics, and dependent on a habitable planet."

Not by chance, the connection between nature and home was an important
insight of the first Greek philosophers who sought to find the key to human
government in biology and physics, namely, the Pythagorean philosophers.
One of them, Philolaus, wrote: "The first thing fitted together, the one [*to
hen*] in the center of the sphere, is called the hearth [*Hestia*]" (Diel Kranz 7
[B91]). Here the "home" or "hearth" does not connote the private dominion
where life is safely governed by the master, but it refers to a principle of harmony composed of the unlimited materiality of life (symbolized by the fire)
and the One that is the principle of all limitation: together they generate the
cosmic order as One Hearth that should become the model for all political
order. The human species will be able to find their way back (Gr. *nostos*, from
which some philologists say derives the Greek term *nous*, or mind (Lachterman, 1990) to this One Home as long as it understands, as Walter Benjamin
(1996 [1928]) says:

Technology is the mastery not of nature but of the relation between nature
and humanity. Men as a species completed their development thousands

of years ago, but humanity as a species is just getting started. In technology, a nature is being organized through which mankind's contact with the cosmos takes a new and different form from that which it had in nations and families. . . . Living substance conquers the frenzy of destruction only in the ecstasy of reproduction.

(p. 487)

Economics originally meant the government of the household (*oikos*). One of the most stunning biopolitical consequences of the Covid-19 pandemic, as many economists have noted, is that the lockdown at home has led to a definitive break with the analogy between household debt and public debt that underpinned decades of neoliberal austerity policies (Tooze & Schularick, 2020). If the pandemic forces us into our homes but allows us to consider what is our true "one home," the same necessity to stay at home, like the sword that wounds and heals in one stroke, also freed us from the dogma that considers public debt as if it were the sum of debts incurred by households. The home lockdown, paradoxically, has made the *oikos*-nomy into a *political* matter once again. But we do not yet know how different this new "political" approach to economics will be from traditional political economy that Marx had already critiqued. The celerity with which all governments have relinquished all budgetary and fiscal restraint, which neoliberals considered the real standard of legitimacy, is indeed quite revolutionary in undoing the neoliberal imperative to privatize debt and risk. However, it is also reactionary in so far as it brings back the old faith in the providential state as the lender of last resort and ultimate social safety net. The risk associated with recurring to this medieval faith in the "immortal" nature of the fisc is that such economic-theological belief underwrites an identification of sovereign power with saving power, the myth of the state as God's representative on earth (Kantorowicz, 1997 [1957]). Unscrupulous rulers and investors will, undoubtedly, try not to let this "good crisis go to waste". The rest of us need to consider that One Health and One Home also entails One Humanity, whose dignity stands above the sovereignty of states and whose worth is beyond market-allocated price. There is no doubt that a pandemic is a brutal way to reveal the vulnerability of all living human specimens. The protection offered by an immortal corporation like the state promises us a degree of invulnerability. Yet what we really hope for in times like these is not the invulnerability of our finite, mortal specimen lives but to experience the life that is eternal.[1] This can only be attained by living up to the humanity in us and to the harmony or law of nature above us.

Note

1 "Yet it is impossible that we should remember that we existed before our body, since neither can there be any traces of this in the body nor can eternity be defined by time, or be in any way related to time. Nevertheless, we feel and experience that we are eternal." Ethics V, P 23, Sch. in (Spinoza, 2002), commented in Vatter (2011).

References

Agamben, G. (2020a). The invention of an epidemic. *European Journal of Psychoanalysis*. www.journal-psychoanalysis.eu/coronavirus-and-philosophers/

Agamben, G. (2020b). Reflections on the plague. *European Journal of Psychoanalysis*. www.journal-psychoanalysis.eu/reflections-on-the-plague/

Benjamin, W. (1996). To the planetarium. In *Benjamin studies* (p. 487). Harvard University Press. (Original work published 1928)

Benvenuto, S. (2020, March 23). Estizzazione: La nostra vita dopo il coronavirus [Estizzazione: Our life after coronavirus]. *Doppiozero*. www.doppiozero.com/materiali/estizzazione-la-nostra-vita-dopo-il-coronavirus

Butler, J. (2020, March 30). *Capitalism has its limits*. www.versobooks.com/blogs/4603-capitalism-has-its-limits

Kantorowicz, E. H. (1997). *The king's two bodies: A study in medieval political theology*. Princeton University Press. (Original work published 1957)

Lachterman, D. (1990). Noos and nostos: The Odyssey and the origins of Greek philosophy. In J. F. Mattei (Ed.), *La naissance de la raison en Grèce* (pp. 33–39). PUF.

Lemm, V. (2020). *Homo natura: Nietzsche, philosophical anthropology and biopolitics*. Edinburgh University Press.

Monbiot, G. (2020, March 25). Covid-19 is nature's wake-up call to complacent civilisation. *The Guardian*. www.theguardian.com/commentisfree/2020/mar/25/covid-19-is-natures-wake-up-call-to-complacent-civilisation

One Health. (n.d.). www.fao.org/asiapacific/perspectives/one-health/en/

Schmitt, C. (2014). The planetary tension between orient and occident and the opposition between land and sea. *Política Común*, *5*. https://doi.org/10.3998/pc.12322227.0005.011[1]

Spinoza, B. (2002). *The complete works* (S. Shirley, Trans.). Hackett.

Tooze, A., & Schularick, M. (2020, March 25). The shock of coronavirus could split the EU – unless nations share the burden. *The Guardian*. www.theguardian.com/commentisfree/2020/mar/25/shock-coronavirus-split-europe-nations-share-burden

Vatter, M. (2011). Eternal life and biopower. *The New Centennial Review*, *10*(3), 217–249.

Žižek, S. (2020, February 27). Coronavirus is "Kill Bill"-esque blow to capitalism and could lead to reinvention of communism. *RT*. www.rt.com/op-ed/481831-coronavirus-kill-bill-capitalism-communism/

14 The Italian laboratory

Rethinking debt in viral times

Elettra Stimilli
March 29, 2020

Once again Italy has become the testing ground for processes and experiences that have become global. The coronavirus has given rise to a completely novel phenomenon, which is not just a political or economic event in itself but a pandemic whose ferocity and rapid transmission requires extraordinary measures. Italy has become the avant-garde of the West, the first to be fully implicated after the initial outbreak in China. Italy is the "laboratory" of the West.

It is no surprise that this absolutely exceptional situation has reignited the Italian debate concerning the "state of exception." Giorgio Agamben reignited this debate with the publication of his article "The State of Exception Has Provoked an Unmotivated Emergency" in the Italian newspaper *Il Manifesto* on February 26 (2020a). He has since reasserted and defended his initial statements in a short piece titled "Clarifications" (Agamben, 2020b). In his criticism of the government's drastic containment measures, Agamben reintroduces, with a particular vehemence and determination, his famous critique of the paradigm of the state of exception. The greatest danger today, he argues, is not the virus itself but the fact that politicians are exploiting this situation in order introduce heightened security measures and deploy a range of exceptional technologies of power. These measures and technologies will be soon regularized by the "invention" of a new paradigm of power: pandemic domination. This is a point he further clarifies in his more recent French interview in *Le Monde* (Agamben, 2020c).

Given Agamben's international role in our contemporary cultural spheres, the complexity of our moment, and the conditions in Italy right now, it is paramount that we move beyond the specificities of Agamben's words and reflect on the reception of his critical intervention – a litmus test for the scope and range of our public debate, which is decisive at this moment. One cannot help but notice that so many interventions, despite their critical intentions, tend to treat the disciplinary operations and social control measures as the effects of a more complex process, which is currently being communicated through the coronavirus. Thus, it is necessary that we rethink "bare life," which Agamben continues to refer to as that form of life that can be sacrificed for the cause of mere survival. But what are the stakes for the survival of bare life which is vulnerable?[1]

What this crisis is making clearly evident is the fact that vulnerable lives are not merely "naked," because vulnerable lives are always involved in conditions where they are, at the very "least," reproduced and taken care of. This reproductive and care work, always adjacent to survival, is completely negated by Agamben's theory. What is also emerging is the fact the virus cannot be treated as a purely biological phenomenon, unrelated to the context in which it is developing. We cannot forget how global capitalism has contributed to the ongoing ecological destruction. Environmental diversity and differences that would have previously interrupted the transmission of pathogenetic agents have been severely eroded. Our globalized modes have facilitated an ease of movement that Covid-19 has taken advantage of. Not only can pathogenetic agents be diffused today at speeds previously unimaginable, but because they can also mutate and adapt at such accelerated rates, it gives rise to more aggressive and lethal variations.

If it is possible to think that the extraction and exploitative processes that had up until yesterday seemed unstoppable have come to a halt, even if perhaps for just a brief moment in these days of a general blockade – as described in a fascinating and imaginary "virus monologue" ["What the Virus Said" (2020)] – then we must also move beyond our obsession with the restrictions of our liberties (which are nothing but the other side of lost privileges) and turn our attention to what is awaiting us, or rather what can be expected, when everything starts up again.

Italy alongside nine other European countries – amongst which France and the more indebted states of Spain and Greece stand out – have requested a "powerful, cohesive, and timely" financial/economic response from Europe. It is difficult to shake the fear of finding ourselves right back in the conditions that arose when we originally made concessions under the guise of "budget flexibility": expanding our balance sheets by resorting to the market with the issuing of further debt. Countries that spend a lot of money today are at risk of finding themselves powerless against speculative assaults tomorrow. Until recently, the only certainty in Italy was the Save States Fund, or the European Bank loans to states, which would in exchange lead to accepting "blood, sweat, and tears" reforms. Even in our current circumstances the longstanding divisions in the European Union continue to thrive: the northern states (especially Germany and the Netherlands) versus the Mediterranean states that are frightened by the prospect of becoming another Greece 2015. But there are changes as well. Some of the very Northern Axis states that took part in the 2015 Greek debt shenanigans, such as France, now find themselves asking for "solidarity measures" in order to manage this current crisis alongside other indebted states. No one wants to sign a memorandum of understanding in order to save their own public finances, particularly those that have already experienced these memorandums at their own expense. Is it possible to imagine that Europe, and particularly Germany and the Netherlands, have rethought their positions? Is it really possible to imagine that the coronavirus has put a halt to those mechanisms that delivered Europe into its so-called sovereign debt crisis after the financial crackdown of 2007–2008?

In his article published in the *Financial Times* on March 25, Mario Draghi (2020) stressed that we are "faced with unforeseen circumstances," however "the loss of income is not the fault of any of those who suffer from it" (as was argued during the sovereign debt crisis). Recalling the European suffering in the 1920s, he adds, "a change of mindset is as necessary in this crisis as it would be in times of war." On the one hand, his proposed solution actually sounds like a radical shift. On the other hand, it mirrors the increases in public debt, only this time shared by Europe and financed by taxes. A problem of correspondence will become an issue between the introduction of massive liquidity and the exorbitant devaluation of capital: no real value can correspond to the currency issued. This same issue arises during a period war, and as with wartimes past it has also precipitated periods of reconstruction.

At this point, however, it is worth questioning whether today it is necessary to elicit war discourse, as Macron is fond of doing, to deploy an army against the virus, or as with Putin, who have joined efforts to send military troops to Italy in the form of humanitarian aid. What we are faced with every day while trapped in our homes is in reality, especially when thought about seriously, not simply an enemy but the proliferation of a life whose reproduction has been somehow facilitated by us. Rather than automatically, and presumably unconsciously, erecting security regimes by declaring states of emergency in the guise of self-defense, it is time to recognize that spaces of political autonomy are also emerging, promoted by those who are looking for a voice, which is being demonstrated in our current public debates.

Today, in our suspended existence, together in fear and pain, we are perhaps also experiencing the profound force of singular lives. Due to many factors, that which we are living is not just a natural catastrophe, a state of exception, or a world war. We need new words. If our inescapable individual competition has prevented us up to this point from understanding, confining us to lonely and indebted existence, perhaps only collective cooperation will enable us to invent new forms of living together (*convivenza*). No power from above can function in the battle against the virus without a mobilization from below that unleashes the strength available to everyone. We must find a collective mode that cares for and transforms the fears that form an integral part of our lives into a powerful expression of our voices and bodies, instead of paralyzing us in face of paranoid scenes of the phenomenon.

Translated from the Italian by Greg Bird

Note

1 This is a question I raised in an earlier paper, "Being in Common at a Distance," that was published in a special issue of *Topia* on this pandemic edited by Greg Bird and Penelope Ironstone. Other essays in this collection, such as Greg Bird's "Biomedical Apparatuses or Conviviality" and Stuart Murray's "COVID-19: Crisis, Critique, and the Limits of What We Can Hear," also deal with the relationship between structural vulnerability and bare life.

References

Agamben, G. (2020a, February 26). Lo stato d'eccezione provocato da un'emergenza immotivata [The state of exception has provoked an unmotivated emergency]. *Il Manifesto*. https://ilmanifesto.it/lo-stato-deccezione-provocato-da-unemergenza-immotivata/

Agamben, G. (2020b, March 17). Chiarimenti [Clarifications]. *Quodlibet*. www.quodlibet.it/giorgio-agamben-chiarimenti?fbclid=IwAR2_SmWYbFJTk75vv515vJ1_Xej1uBeL-RLhUgAiHUxFkJZiwitmZZ-q9eY

Agamben, G. (2020c, March 25). L'épidémie montre clairement que l'état d'exception est devenu la condition normale [Normalizing the state of exception under the Covid-19 epidemic]. *Le Monde*. www.lemonde.fr/idees/article/2020/03/24/giorgio-agamben-l-epidemie-montre-clairement-que-l-etat-d-exception-est-devenu-la-condition-normale_6034245_3232.html

Draghi, M. (2020, March 25). We face a war against coronavirus and must mobilise accordingly. *The Financial Times*. www.ft.com/content/c6d2de3a-6ec5-11ea-89df-41bea055720b

"What the Virus Said" (2020, May 16). *lundimatin#*. https://lundi.am/What-the-virus-said

15 *Vitam instituere*

Roberto Esposito
March 26, 2020

If I had to name the task that the coronavirus entrusts us with, I would use the ancient Latin expression *vitam instituere*. Without retracing its history – it is a passage from Demosthenes, quoted by the Roman jurist Marcianus in the *Digest* – we may focus on its most current meaning. At a time when human life appears to be threatened and overpowered by death, our common effort can only be that of 'establishing' it again and again. What else, after all, is life if not this continuous 'establishment', the capacity to create ever new meanings. It is in this sense that Hannah Arendt, and before her Augustine, said that we, mankind, constitute a beginning because our first action is to come into the world, starting something that was not before. This first beginning was followed by another, a further founding act, constituted by language – the French psychoanalyst Pierre Legendre called it a second birth. It is from this birth that the city and political life originate, providing biological life with a historical horizon. This horizon is not in contrast with the world of nature, rather it traverses it in all its extension. The space of *logos*, and then of *nomos*, however autonomous in its wealth of configurations, has never become separate from that of *bios*. On the contrary, their relationship has become increasingly closer, to the point it is impossible to talk about politics by removing it from the sphere in which life is generated.

The first birth announces the second one in that the latter is rooted in the first. For this reason, it is not possible for human beings to abstain from establishing life, for it is life that has instituted these same human beings by placing them in a common world. In this sense, human life cannot be reduced to simple survival – to 'bare life', we may say, quoting Benjamin. Having been established from the very beginning, our life never coincides with mere biological matter – even when it is crushed against it. And also in this case, perhaps especially in this case, life as such reveals a way of being that, however deformed, violated, trampled on, remains such – a form of life. What gives it this formal character – something other than mere biology – is its belonging to a historical context, constituted by social, political and symbolic relations. What establishes us from the beginning, what we ourselves continually establish, is this symbolic pattern within which everything we do acquires meaning and significance for us and for others.

It is precisely this pattern of common relations that the coronavirus threatens to break. Not only the first type of life, but also the second – the social character of our relationship with others. Clearly, in order to express itself, the latter requires to be alive. The term 'survival' bears no reductive connotation. On the contrary, the problem of *conservatio vitae* is at the heart of classical and modern culture. It resonates in the Christian conception of sacred life, as in the great political philosophical tradition inaugurated by Hobbes. The first task this wretched virus entrusts us with, in its deadly challenge, is to stay alive. What is more, by defending this first life, we must also defend the second life, established life, which is, for this reason, the one able to establish and create new meaning. Therefore, at a time when we are doing all that is in our power to stay alive, as is understandable, we cannot renounce the second life – life with others, for others, through others. This is not, however, allowed; in fact it is, rightly and logically, forbidden.

To consider this sacrifice as unbearable, when there are those who are risking their lives in hospitals to save ours, is not only offensive; it is ridiculous. In no way does this diminish established life. Nor does it diminish the need to continue, despite everything, and even more so at a time when social relations are wounded, to live in common. Also alone. Giving a common sense to this aloneness. It is, in fact, precisely that which today connects us to others. To all others – at present half of humanity, perhaps in a month's time it will be the whole of humanity. After all, distance itself is also a profoundly human dimension – the same way closeness is, from which it derives its meaning. Not only by contrast – 'individual' has never been the mere opposite of 'social', it is in turn a social construct. Today this symbolic link between distance and proximity – the symbol is precisely the figure articulating it – acquires even greater importance. In times of pandemic, human beings are united by a common distance. Yet also this is a way – at present a necessary one – of establishing life, of defending it from the blind force that threatens to devour it.

**Translated from the Italian
by Emma Catherine Gainsforth**

16 Communovirus

Jean-Luc Nancy
March 24, 2020

An Indian friend of mine tells me that back home they talk about the 'communovirus'. How could we not have thought of that already? It's so obvious! And what an admirable and complete ambivalence: a virus coming from communism, a virus that communizes us. That is much more fertile than the derisory 'corona', which evokes old monarchical or imperial histories. And 'communo' is good for dethroning 'corona', if not decapitating it.

This is what it seems to be doing in its first meaning, since it comes from the largest country in the world whose regime is officially communist. It is not just officially so: as President Xi Jinping has said, its management of the viral epidemic demonstrates the superiority of the 'socialist system with Chinese characteristics'. Though communism consists essentially in the abolition of private property, Chinese communism has consisted, for many years now, in a careful combination of collective (or state) property and private property (apart from land ownership).[1]

As we know, this combination has led to remarkable growth in China's economic and technical capacities and its global role. It is still too soon to know how to designate the society produced by this combination: in what sense is it communist and in what sense has it introduced the virus of individual competition, even its ultraliberal extreme? For the time being, the Covid-19 virus has enabled China to demonstrate the effectiveness of the collective and state aspect of its system. This effectiveness has proved itself to the point that China is now coming to the aid of Italy and France.

Of course, there is no shortage of comments on the enhanced authoritarian power that the Chinese state is currently enjoying. In fact, it is just as if the virus appeared at the right time to shore up official communism. What is irksome is that in this way the meaning of the word 'communism' gets ever more blurred – and it was already uncertain.

Marx wrote very precisely that private property had meant the disappearance of collective property, and that both would be replaced in due course by what he called 'individual property'. By this he did not mean goods owned individually (i.e. private property) but the possibility for individuals to become properly themselves. One could say: to realize themselves. Marx did not have the time or means to take this line of thought further. But we can at least recognize that it already opens up a convincing – if very indeter-minate – perspective on a 'communist' proposal. 'To realize oneself' does not mean acquiring material or symbolic goods: it means becoming real, effective, existing in a unique way.

We need then to dwell on the second meaning of 'communovirus'. In fact, the virus actually does communize us. It essentially puts us on a basis of equal-ity, bringing us together in the need to make a common stand. That this must involve the isolation of each of us is simply a paradoxical way of experiencing our community. We can only be unique together. This is what makes for our most intimate community: the shared sense of our uniqueness.

Today, and in every way, we are reminded of our togetherness, interde-pendence and solidarity. Testimonies and initiatives in this sense are coming from all sides. If we add to this the decline in air pollution due to the reduc-tion of transport and industry, some people already anticipate with delight the overthrow of techno-capitalism. We should not scoff at this fragile euphoria but rather ask ourselves how far we can better understand the nature of our community.

Solidarity is called for and activated on a large scale, but the overall media landscape is dominated by the expectation of state welfare – which Emmanuel Macron took the opportunity to celebrate. Instead of confining ourselves, we feel confined primarily by force, even if for the sake of our own welfare. We experience isolation as a deprivation, even when it is a protection.

In a way, this is an excellent catch-up session: it is true that we are not soli-tary animals. It is true that we need to meet up, have a drink and visit. Besides, the sudden rise in phone calls, emails and other social flows shows a pressing need, a fear of losing contact.

Does this mean we are in a better position to reflect on this community? The problem is that the virus is still its main representative, that between the surveillance model and the welfare model, only the virus remains as a common property.

If this is the case, we will make no progress in understanding what transcend-ing both collective and private property could mean. That is to say, transcend-ing both property in general and what it designates in terms of the possession of an object by a subject. The characteristic of the 'individual', to speak as Marx did, is to be incomparable, incommensurable and unassimilable – even to themselves. It is not to possess 'goods'. It is to be a unique, exclusive possibil-ity of realization, whose exclusive uniqueness is realized, by definition, only between all and with all – also against all or in spite of all, but always in rela-tion and exchange (communication). This is a 'value' that is neither one of the general equivalent (money) nor, therefore, one of an extorted 'surplus-value', but a value that cannot be measured in any way.

Are we capable of thinking in such a difficult – and even dizzying – fashion? It is good that the 'communovirus' forces us to ask ourselves this question. For it is only on this condition that it is worthwhile, in the end, working to eliminate it. Otherwise we will end up back at the starting point. We will be relieved but should be prepared for other pandemics.

Translated from the French
by David Fernbach

Note

1 The published text has here 'individual property', which seems accidental in view of the author's use of the term below (Trans.).

17 Satanization of man

The pandemic and the wound of narcissism

Sergio Benvenuto
June 1, 2020

In many cultures once referred to as "primitive", it is inconceivable for someone to die a natural death. For example, among the Jivaros of South America, even if a person is 80 years old and dies in her own bed, it will be taken for granted that she was victim of black magic and that someone wished to harm her. Hence the person responsible for the death has to be found and punished.

It would be naïve to think that it is merely a question of superstitious primitive beliefs: the logic of the scapegoat – seeking a human fault in everything that is natural – applies to us hyper-industrialized moderns too. So among the several theories on the origins of the coronavirus pandemic that are flourishing, some point a stern finger at super-industrialization: pollution, the greenhouse effect, hyperbolized urbanization, the reduction of biodiversity, and so forth. In other words, Man is the true cause of disasters, not too different from Rousseau's arguments after the catastrophic earthquake that struck Lisbon in 1755: nature is in itself benign. It is human beings who create the ills that sap them. Our culture digs our grave. Another inverse theory is that, unsurprisingly, coronavirus first appeared in China, where promiscuity between animals and humans is highest. Besides, Chinese people eat bats (but it's been established that before the epidemic there were no bats on sale in Wuhan). The *spillover* theory (Quammen, 2012) of viruses being passed on from one species to another is a very serious one – but it's being used to stigmatize "those primitives", the Chinese.

The theories that accuse human beings – *always*, whatever happens – as the primary cause of their own woes follow the same logic as that of the Jivaros, who refuse to accept the idea of a *natural* death without human intervention. The only difference is that the human causes no longer concern a single individual, but human beings as a whole. Not just *a* man, but *Man* is charged with being the perpetrator of the blights afflicting humankind.

The truth is that epidemics have always existed and always will – simple and disappointing, but true. Despite all of our technology, we are still prey to nature. The Black Death, which annihilated half the population of Europe in the 14th century, was not of course an effect of industrialization but of an absolutely natural mutation that Darwinism has made perfectly intelligible. Viruses mutate far more quickly than evolved animal species, which is why we have to find a new influenza vaccine every year: between one winter and the next, the virus species will have mutated. So today, with electronic society in full expansion, we have to rely on the same epidemic containment techniques used thousands of years ago: not having any specific medications, all we can do is isolate people from each other as much as possible. This was not done in 1918 with the Spanish flu because the world was still at war and the epidemic was underestimated, and the death toll was between 20 and 100 million (according to the calculation methods of the time).

Today many talk of the Anthropocene epoch, and it is true that *Homo sapiens* are modifying – for worse – the conditions of the planet. I am the last to underestimate the threats posed by pollution, by the greenhouse effect and by the reduction of biodiversity – but human destructive power should not be overestimated either. We bring about and are subject to essential events just like at the dawn of *Homo sapiens*: we reproduce in the majority of cases through coitus, our children are neotenic, they are subject to a very long infancy, sooner or later they die, they are occasionally mown down by epidemics: this is the way it will always be. Blaming humans for every ill is the other side of the divinization of Man (which dates back to Pascal) that many contemporary philosophies have condemned: if one thinks that humans are ultimately as powerful as God, it will also be thought that they may possess the same evil omnipotence as Satan. But man is neither God nor Satan.

The search for a human scapegoat can take on primitive, crude and vulgar forms in an uncultivated population and refined, philosophical, sophisticated ones among well-read minorities. But they are both varieties of the same prejudice.

A perfect example of the coarsest form was expressed by President Trump, who immediately found "the culprit" of the Covid-19 epidemic in China, first calling the coronavirus "the Chinese Virus".

According to some slightly more sophisticated theories (notably, those of Nobel laureate Luc Montagnier), Covid-19 is not the result of a mere Darwinian mutation among viruses but the effect of genetic engineering. The virus was supposedly created in Chinese laboratories, perhaps to find a vaccine against HIV, and then the biologists there lost control of it (a thesis endorsed by Trump as well). Many find the hypothesis attractive because, in this case too, the pandemic is seen as the effect of human technology.

Some more sophisticated theories blame Man, society, our ideological system and so on as the cause of the pandemic or of its amplified impact. In particular, we have the theses upheld by the famous Italian philosopher Giorgio Agamben.

In a series of articles, Agamben (2020a, 2020b, 2020c) first argued that the coronavirus pandemic was an invention by political power to impose a "state of exception", a subject he has been fond of for decades (Agamben, 2005). At first it sounds like a purely denialist thesis that someone could equate to other forms of denialism that are spreading like viruses today: Holocaust denial, climate change denial, denial of the harmlessness of vaccines against childhood diseases and so on. A few days later, Agamben softened his position saying that the political powers took advantage of the pandemic to impose an authoritarian regime limiting individual freedoms – as if political leaders greatly benefited from blocking the productive activities of their respective countries and creating an overwhelming economic crisis.

I do not condemn as heresies all the theses that tend to scale down the actual extent of the pandemic and deny its gravity. Some say, after all, that in many affected countries the average mortality rate during the winter and spring seasons, when the pandemic exploded, was not much higher than in the same period in previous years. And there are other arguments. These are theses I am prepared to confront myself with because they are based on data, statistics and probabilistic forecasting. Data can indeed be interpreted in different ways, but it is something quite different from trying to deny the reach of the epidemic on the basis of conspiratorial theoretical premises according to which political power or capitalism manipulate and subjugate us.

Agamben's position is the extreme pole of that whole host of opinions that consider human beings the fundamental cause of the pandemic.

It is been stressed that the pandemic hit so many countries because capitalism gives a frenetic impulse to mobility (even to migrations, but anti-capitalists do not mention this, because they sympathize with migrants).

The French philosopher Alain Badiou (2020), after specifying that this epidemic is nothing new or extraordinary, adds: "we know that the world market, combined with the existence of vast under-medicalized zones and the lack of global discipline when it comes to the necessary vaccinations, inevitably produces serious and devastating epidemics." And he goes on to say that "the planetary diffusion of this point of origin [Wuhan]" is "borne by the capitalist world market and its reliance on rapid and incessant mobility." He is hinting that epidemics due to the worldwide (capitalist) market are completely different from those that spread in pre-capitalist times! This is of course quite absurd. I wonder what the link is between the existence of medically under-served zones (which exist of course, especially in Africa) and the origin and spread of Covid-19. What is puzzling is that Wuhan is by no means an under-medicalized zone (in fact, the Chinese response to the epidemic was highly effective) and the virus first spread in the wealthiest parts of the world, where the health system is quite efficient. In fact, Marxist philosophers *must* be evoking all of these problems (the capitalist market, poor areas, etc.) as if reciting a litany, as a conditioned reflex, even if these problems have no clear connection with other kinds of ills we are dealing with.

It is true that many of the worst-hit areas in various countries (Lombardy, New York, etc.) are the most *mobile*. But what model of society *other* than capitalism do these thinkers have in mind? One with limited trade, exchanges and transportation, closed like medieval Japan? Is this the kind of post-capitalist society they are suggesting instead of capitalism?

Badiou, like others, is evidently mixing up *modernization* and *capitalism*. By modernization I mean the expansion of technology and the application of scientific discoveries within society, a process that has historically coincided with the development of capitalism but does not necessarily identify with the latter. I wonder whether the anti-capitalism of so many actually conceals simply a rejection of modern technological society, a somewhat regressive aspiration.

Fortunately, until now the poorest countries of Africa seem to have been hit less than rich industrialized countries (I do not know if that will be still true when these lines are published). Had the opposite happened, I can almost hear the chorus of many intellectuals: immediately they would have ranted about how this disparity in infections was an effect of capitalism, establishing a close relationship between the virus and under-development, and so on.

The limit of every ideology — therefore also of the neo-Marxist or neo-anarchist ones I am targeting here — is trying to force anything that happens into a predetermined framework. Of course, theories are indispensable to sim-plify the chaotic complexity of the world, but they always risk being a bed of Procrustes onto which reality is forced. Some refuse to admit that reality can refute or relativize their theories and will always come up with ways to find their ideas confirmed. Many academic "critical theories" lack any critical spirit.

An epidemic, whether it was the plague, or cholera, and so on, used to be interpreted as a divine punishment for human sins. Today, instead, an intel-lectual elite interprets an epidemic as a punishment that human beings inflict upon themselves. Many think that "nature rebels against humans". Nature has taken the place of God as the punisher. But for others, *Homo sapiens* ruin them-selves for the sin of having generated capitalistic societies.

In fact, in the last century a process of divinizing the human being has replaced God. Secularization, taken for granted today, is a divinization of the human. "God is dead", Nietzsche affirmed, and we humans had killed him. But the death of God leaves *the place* of divinity vacant, which tends to be occupied more and more by Man. The human being wants to become what this divine being was: omnipotent. Today science and technology are the human activities that seem more than any other to promise the divine elevation of man.

But every divinization always produces, as its inevitable shadow, the antiph-rasis of diabolical power. Every God leads to the emergence of its counterpart demons. If God created the world and the world is full of evil, then there must be a counter-God somewhere. It may not be omnipotent like God, but it cer-tainly is extremely powerful. It was in fact the counter-God who humanized Adam and Eve, tearing them away from their subdued bliss. If human beings replace God, then they can replace Satan too. Divinized human beings self-produce their own diabolization.

But how do we reconcile this process of divinization of man that seems to mark secularized (i.e. Godless) modernity with the actual *contents* of scientific knowledge, which instead drastically scales down the role of *Homo* in the uni-verse? Freud spoke of three fundamental narcissistic wounds inflicted on man in recent centuries: Copernicanism, Darwinism and psychoanalysis. Copernicus displaced the Earth from the central position of the Ptolemaic universe. Darwin shattered the belief of an essential difference between human beings and other animals. Freud himself inflicted the third narcissistic blow by saying that the ego is not a master in its own home.

Science actually shows us the extent of our human irrelevance in the universe. Yet science, hailed as our new divinity, is invoked as a mark of our overwhelming superiority over all other animals. So, has modernity, from Copernicus onwards, been a narcissistic debasement of the human being, or its elevation to a sort of god?

The truth is that these wounds of human narcissism posited by Freud in turn inflate human narcissism: the more human beings recognize themselves as marginal and random, the more the idea of their desperate might emerges as a form of compensation. Our admittance of irrelevance – "we live in a fair to middling planet in a marginal part of our galaxy" – becomes our pride, the compost of our arrogance: we are capable of not being anthropocentric! "We're the only animals who can look at the world not just from *our* point of view!" But this is not true – even science is anthropocentric. This is where most of the drama of modern thought lies.

Anthropologists tell us that many primitive cultures call themselves "human beings" tout court, as if all other cultures were not human. In this way, these scholars praise themselves as non-ethnocentric, in contrast to the primitive peoples they study, thus affirming obliquely an extraordinary superiority to these peoples. It is the *double bind* Lévi-Strauss ran into when he said: "The barbarian is, first and foremost, the man who believes in barbarism!" But, as many believe that barbarians do of course exist, then barbarism really does exist!

In actual fact, science does not realize – as it is not its job to do so – that what it knows and discovers about the universe will always be a *human point of view*. Objectivity, which is a great ideal, is always a relative quality: the world we know is ultimately the one we need. Philosophical pragmatism said precisely this: that at the end of the day only that which is useful is real for human beings. But instead of being condemned as a limit of humans, as their cage, as a Platonic cave with no way out, this is extolled as the prodigious anthropocentrism of human beings.

References

Agamben, G. (2005). *State of exception*. University of Chicago Press.

Agamben, G. (2020a). Reflections on the plague. *European Journal of Psychoanalysis*. www.journal-psychoanalysis.eu/reflections-on-the-plague/

Agamben, G. (2020b). *Clarifications*. https://medium.com/@ddean3000/clarifications-giorgio-agamben-3f97dc7ed67c

Agamben, G. (2020c). Social distancing. *Autonomies*. http://autonomies.org/2020/04/giorgio-agamben-social-distancing/

Badiou, A. (2020, March 23). *On the epidemic situation*. Verso Books. www.versobooks.com/blogs/4608-on-the-epidemic-situation

Quammen, D. (2012). *Spillover: Animal infections and the next human pandemic*. Norton.

18 A viral revaluation of all values?

Dany Nobus
April 15, 2020

Trying to find a fitting way to begin this brief reflection, I felt like Leonard Cohen when he sat down to write to Marianne Ihlen in his room at the Penn Terminal Hotel in New York City on February 23, 1967. It was the day after his first major performance, in front of 3,000 people, at the Village Theatre, and he conceded that he could hardly write, not because he was in bad shape, but because there was so much or so little to tell (Cohen, 1967). What is there to tell that has not been told numerous times over, about 'unprecedented times', the 'worst peacetime emergency in living times', the 'war against an invisible enemy', 'underlying health conditions', '(the persistent lack of) personal protective equipment', 'social distancing'? What is there to tell when so many words of love, life and death have been blunted by routine usage to such an extent that they cannot possibly be used anymore to relay the singular authenticity of a lived, subjective experience? So much to tell because, quite paradoxically, being in lockdown has sparked a surfeit of new intractable experiences. So little to tell because, quite paradoxically, all distinctly unique, internal experiences have become homogenized in a global, collective experiential lifeworld.

So when and where did it all begin? I cannot remember exactly when I first heard about Covid-19, yet it was undoubtedly quite some time after it was first diagnosed and quite some time before it became almost impossible to hear about anything else. Scientists around the world are reportedly working exceptionally hard to establish the precise origin of the virus in order to be better equipped to prevent the next pandemic (Readfearn, 2020). On the surface, this seems like a perfectly sound kind of reasoning – 'An ounce of prevention is worth a pound of cure', the 13th-century English jurist Henry de Bracton once said – yet unfortunately it also includes a highly uncomfortable truth about the limits and limitations of human life. Were it to be firmly established that patient zero was indeed a Chinese market vendor who unwittingly contracted the virus from an infected bat or pangolin, the only element of truth this zoonotic origin story would contain is that the next pandemic cannot be prevented at all, even if it were driven by an identical viral strain and not to occur for another century or so. Anticipatory and prophylactic health care are not just a function of purportedly evidence-based scientific knowledge about how illnesses happen, diseases spread and epidemics decimate the human population, but also, and much more fundamentally, of how the evidence is manufactured, consolidated and employed. And this assumes that an effective vaccine can be found, which is by no means as indisputable as virologists and epidemiologists would want us to believe. Forty years after the human immunodeficiency virus was properly identified for the first time in humans, and 75 million deaths later, there is still no effective vaccine for HIV.

The intrinsic instability and ineluctable politicization of scientific knowledge is but one of the great many tensions and truths the question of the virus – which should also be understood, here, as a subjective genitive, and thus as the question posed *by* the virus – has magnified and laid bare. To be clear, it is not the viral question in itself which has fully exposed some of the most disturbing aspects of 21st-century life on planet Earth but the socio-political, institutional and personal responses to it, as if the proverbial truth-inducing properties of the freely flowing 'vino' had been ubiquitously replaced with the equally revealing effects of a rapidly replicating virus. If sickness indeed shows us what we are, then what has thus far already been disclosed is that the human and socio-economic cost of the pandemic will be exponentially higher in the neoliberal, individualist West than in the communitarian East. Some autocratic leaders have undoubtedly capitalized on the Chinese relative success in controlling transmission rates in order to legitimize and expand their dictatorial rule, which would be another way to illustrate how 'truth is in the virus', yet the Chinese success story is first and foremost an exemplification of the bankruptcy of the value system underpinning Western political economies. In the weeks leading up to the nationwide lockdown of March 23, 2020, the UK government first entertained the 'scientifically proven' theory of herd immunity, presumably because economic wealth should always take precedence over public health, and then exchanged this approach, allegedly because the 'science' had changed, for an explicit reliance on the general public's individual goodwill to respect the rules of social distancing. Only when it was observed that this individual goodwill was not nearly as reliable as politicians had thought it to be, and that public health (systems) could potentially be put at an even higher risk than under herd immunity strategies, did the perspective change from a recommendation to an imposition. It is important to note, however, that the European (and American) models of containment are not a latter-day replication of the Chinese (and South Korean) approaches, which have gone much further in curtailing individual liberties, and that any such replication, were it to be deemed acceptable, would always already be too little too late. Strange as it may seem, the staggering human and economic cost of the virus in the West is directly proportional to its spurious ideological belief in the productive power of self-governance and individual enterprise.

There are numerous other examples of how the global pandemic has ruthlessly exposed the fissures, fractures and fragilities of human civilization, from hidden or neglected social inequalities to painfully inadequate health care systems, and from the purportedly unassailable health economic principle of cost-effectiveness to personal health as a measure of social status. In this respect, the virus does discriminate, because Black and minority ethnic people are significantly more likely to contract it and subsequently die from Covid-19 than other sections of the population (Lynch, 2020). In this respect, the current global war against the invisible enemy does not just exist in the general population and in hospitals but also (and much more surreptitiously) in the great many public and private care homes for the elderly and other vulnerable citizens. In this respect, working from home to protect oneself, one's neighbors, and the healthcare system is not just a general rule that can be rolled out indiscriminately to everyone (apart from the so-called key workers), but a concrete professional practice whose successful implementation not only depends on the flexibility of the employer and the creativity of the worker, but most crucially on the 'level' of the work undertaken, and thus on social status.

It is far too early to tell whether the pandemic will lead to a complete 'revaluation of all values', along the lines Nietzsche called for, although in his case as a radical alternative to the Christian 'immortal blot on humanity' (Nietzsche, 2005 [1888], p. 66) rather than the equally invincible rise of global capitalism. In a thoughtful piece on the impact of the coronavirus on climate change, which moved far beyond the platitudes of 'nature steadily bouncing back' in the now largely deserted areas of former human pollution, Arthur Wyns, a researcher working for the World Health Organization, recently argued that the pandemic may very well elicit a more profound appreciation of our vulnerabilities and of the global ties that bind us, which may in turn generate a better understanding of the most important threat to our human survival, i.e. the climate crisis (Wyns, 2020). Pessimist as I am, and uplifting as the statement may be, I remain unsure whether this message of hope will come to pass. There is little doubt that Western economies will need a long time to recover from the as yet immeasurable damage that has been inflicted upon all the constitutive organs of its supposedly resilient body. There is little doubt that historical time will be punctuated by a 'before' and an 'after corona', and that our collective memories will be forever tainted by the time when the world stood still. Yet none of this implies that the recovery process will also entail a radical revision of the value systems which, if they cannot be held responsible for a Chinese market vendor interacting with a bat or pangolin, can definitely to some extent be held to account for the ongoing transmission of a lethal virus and the hundreds of thousands of deaths it has carried in its wake. For a viral revaluation of all values to happen, maybe the pandemic will have ended too soon, much like, in Freud's infamous words to his Hungarian colleague Sándor Ferenczi, World War I effectively ended too soon for psychiatry to become de-stabilized and psychoanalysis to benefit from the collapse of its scientific hegemony (Falzeder et al., 1996, p. 311). Maybe in 500 years, historians will look back upon the year 2020 as the beginning of the second Renaissance; maybe in 500 years, 2020 will merely be recorded as an extremely significant yet ultimately controlled disruption in the course of human existence.

References

Cohen, L. (1967). *Letter to Marianne Ihlen of 23 February 1967*. Private Collection.

Falzeder, E., Brabant, E., & Giampieri-Deutsch, P. (Eds.). (1996). *The correspondence of Sigmund Freud and Sándor Ferenczi: Vol. 2: 1914–1919* (P. T. Hoffer, Trans.). Belknap Press of Harvard University Press.

Lynch, C. (2020, April 10). Coronavirus: Black and Hispanic people "twice as likely to die" in US from COVID-19. *Sky News*. Retrieved April 14, 2020, from https://news.sky.com/story/coronavirus-black-and-hispanic-people-twice-as-likely-to-die-in-us-from-covid-19-11971690

Nietzsche, F. (2005). The anti-Christ: A curse on Christianity. In A. Ridley & J. Norman (Eds.), J. Norman (Trans.), *The anti-Christ, Ecce Homo, twilight of the idols, and other writings* (pp. 1–67). Cambridge University Press. (Original work published 1888)

Readfearn, G. (2020, April 27). How did coronavirus start and where did it come from? Was it really Wuhan's animal market? *The Guardian*. Retrieved April 14, 2020, from www.theguardian.com/world/2020/apr/15/how-did-the-coronavirus-start-where-did-it-come-from-how-did-it-spread-humans-was-it-really-bats-pangolins-wuhan-animal-market

Wyns, A. (2020, April 2). *How our responses to climate change and the coronavirus are linked*. World Economic Forum. www.weforum.org/agenda/2020/04/climate-change-coronavirus-linked/

19 Humanity is rediscovering existential solitude, the meaning of limits, and mortality

Julia Kristeva
April 29, 2020

Julia Kristeva:	"We stayed in Paris, but many people from our neighborhood left to spend these days of isolation in other places. So, at 8 pm, when from the balconies comes applause for doctors and nurses, me and my husband (the philosopher Philippe Sollers) bang on pots and pans to make some extra noise." – *Julia Kristeva (this interview was conducted over the phone).*
C.D.S.:	(*Corriere della Sera*): Along with outbursts of solidarity and moments of communion from the balconies, social isolation has also begun to provoke jealousies and aggression. There is hatred expressed against those who have managed to reach their summer houses or against those who are suspected of doing a little too much jogging. Is the coronavirus jeopardizing social relations?
Julia Kristeva:	It is curious how before the pandemic the word "viral" was already being used a lot and for quite some time. "Viral" reactions were already part of our hyperconnected economic and political reality. Everything that proceeds by contagion, precipitation, and then, after a sparkling beginning linked to pleasure, culminates in a deadly explosion. "Virality" is part of our environment, for example where social media exalt themselves only to mistreat and destroy. In the behaviors that you are citing, there is something viral, but we have seen it in action before too: in the *gilets jaunes*, a movement that urged people to rise up, but also destroyed, in the *black bloc* that were plundering the streets of Paris. The acceleration of our civilization had already arrived at a viral stage, and today this metaphor overwhelms us and enters into the real, because it is an internal as well as an external menace – perhaps we do not have strong enough immune defenses and the danger is therefore also inside of us. Some have the virus maybe without even knowing it, but will survive, while others will die. This allows us to ask ourselves questions about the world in which we live, its failings and

about that which we do not succeed in thinking. Beginning with Europe.

C.D.S.:   How are you evaluating the role of Europe at this stage?

Julia Kristeva: I am European and in the book on Dostoevsky that I just published, I look for the European and modern dimension. I see Europe everywhere and I want to sustain it, even though it is traversing many difficulties and finds itself in a moment of chaos. But the virus has shown that this Europe is not only a market without a clear political vision, without defense mechanisms, incapable of rethinking our great common culture, but that this Europe is also demonstrating an absolutely frightening healthcare incapacity. The need for medical equipment has been severely underestimated both in Italy and in France, and this seems to me a refusal to think about the fragility of the human species. And this can bring us to the plane of individual behaviors. From the metaphor of the viral, we move on to the reality of the viral, to what the epidemic reveals about the individual, about today's globalized man.

C.D.S.:   What are the characteristics of this globalized man?

Julia Kristeva: I see three: solitude experienced as loneliness, an intolerance of limits, and repression of mortality.

C.D.S.:   How is loneliness manifested?

Julia Kristeva: I am struck by our contemporary incapacity to be alone. All this hyper-connected exaltation makes us live in isolation in front of screens. This has not abolished loneliness, but has ensconced it in the social media, has compressed it in messages and data. People already devastated by loneliness find themselves alone today, because although they have words, signs, icons, they have lost the flesh of words, sensations, sharing, tenderness, duty towards the other, care for the other. We give the flesh of words as a sacrificial offering to the virus and to malady, but we were already orphans of that human dimension that is shared passion.

C.D.S.:   So the quarantine reveals a state that was already present?

Julia Kristeva: Yes. All of a sudden we realize that we are alone and that we have lost touch with our inner core. We are slaves of the screens that have not at all abolished loneliness but have only absorbed it. This is where the recent anxiety and anger are coming from.

C.D.S.:   You are a psychoanalyst. Are you still holding sessions these days?

Julia Kristeva: Yes – and now I will allow myself to preach for my own parish as the saying goes – I was afraid that my patients would not want to continue, but instead no, on the contrary. In our sessions of telephone isolation, as I call them, even without the physical presence of the analyst, we call each other, leave the phone open, stretch out and remain in session, and there come moments of archaic collapse: the cancer of one's own mother reappears, an abandonment one suffered in childhood, the hardships of a daughter. Things that we had not been able to speak about before, now get confronted with dedication, as if the danger forced us to expel our deepest pain. These days, through the telephone, we manage to touch something "nuclear": certain defenses fall down, we bare ourselves with a new sincerity.

C.D.S.: Why is it happening precisely now?

Julia Kristeva: Because the epidemic forces us to confront the other two problems that I mentioned before, besides the question of solitude: limits and mortality. The current situation is making us realize that life is a continual survival because there are limits, obligations, vulnerabilities – dimensions of life that are quite present in all religions, but which the current humanism tends to efface. In the same way, we tend to expel from ourselves the question of mortality, the greatest limit that exists and which is part of nature and of life.

C.D.S.: Is the repression of mortality a recent phenomenon?

Julia Kristeva: Since the Renaissance we have regarded mortality as a matter for religion. It was up to the priests to take care of it. We find it in philosophers, in Hegel and Heidegger, but mortality is absent from common, popular, mediatic discourse. We prefer to forget about it. We might take care of the elderly, but we do not confront the fact that death is within us, in apoptosis, which is the continuous process of death and regeneration of the cells, even in this very moment as I am speaking to you. This new virus makes us face the fact that death plays an integral part in the process of life. Art and literature, I am thinking of Proust and Bataille for example, have reflected on these topics: the very act of writing constitutes a confrontation with death, but the most widespread, mediatic, sensationalist attitude towards the human usually avoids this dimension.

C.D.S.: Do you think that the epidemic will change our perspective on things?

Julia Kristeva: It could influence our family relations, between parents and children, prompt us to rethink consumerism, the obsession with travel, that political fever inspired by slogans like "work more in order to earn more," competitiveness displayed like glitter. I am not proposing a cult of melancholy, but a reevaluation of life as a whole, starting with everyone's vulnerability with regard to pleasure and sexuality.

C.D.S.: What do you mean by a cult of melancholy to be avoided?

Julia Kristeva: I am not proposing becoming imprisoned in finitude and in our limits, but only remaining aware of them, considering mortality as part of life. In every religion, there is the element of purification: one needs to wash oneself, one should not touch this or that, and there are prohibitions. These are superstitions and they become obsessive cults, but we can still take into account this tradition, criticize it, rethink it, but also preserve the sense of precaution, the preoccupation with others and their weaknesses, the awareness of the finitude of life. We can become more prudent, perhaps more tender, and in this way also more resilient, resistant. Life is a permanent survival. We have all survived. Let's remember that. It is a question of behavior, of personal ethics.

C.D.S.:   In the end, are you an optimist?

Julia Kristeva: I would say an energetic pessimist. I feel I have experienced three wars: I was a baby during the Second World War, then there was the Cold War and my exile even though gilded, and now there is the viral war. Perhaps this has prepared me to speak about survival. We are ready for a new art of living that will not be tragic, but rather will be complex and demanding.

20 A flight indestinate

Divya Dwivedi
May 5, 2020

Today satellites make us the "watchers from the sky" of the mass graves wherever the speed of Covid-19 related deaths has outstripped the speed of medical and funerary care. In our confinements, the news websites and social media have become our apertures into extraordinary burial sites: remote islands and refrigerator trucks. Unlike what Agamben seems to suggest, this experience of incomplete ritualistic mourning is not new (Agamben, 2020a). After all, man was not set into civilization in an instant through a singular act of the "heavens." Through Thucydides's (1998 [431 BCE]) accounts we know that epidemics in the ancient times too gave rise to such a situation: "All the funeral customs they had previously observed were thrown into confusion. . . . Many of them . . . turned to shameless burial methods. . . . No fear of the gods or law of man was a deterrent" [II.53–54] (pp. 100–101).

Burials and laments were never and still are not the mere symbolic form of "respect." Nor are they a permanent metaphor of returning to dust. Handling the dead has always been a part of the arrangements for the circulations of health and sickness among the living and the non-living, the soils, the plants and the animals, including the human animal. Every once in a while, as the components of this circulation change and outgrow each other, the arrangements must be changed and tended.

Today, separated from their dead for the sake of their own health, thousands of people mourn in the company of strangers via tele-technologies. The journalists of the world have assumed a polynomial existence, functioning all at once as witnesses, postmen, confessors, runners of meagre rations. The very vocation of the lament is borne no longer by religions (which in the best instances today are feeding and sheltering the unclaimed living). Instead, the lament is now raised for the living by nurses and doctors who plead with the protestors who oppose lockdowns.

Health advisors and relief groups plead with governments to sagaciously plan both the confinement and the traffic in necessary supplies. Researchers plead with everyone whom they can reach to discard superstitions and rumors, to heed the humility of reason and of established facts. These are today's blind seers who know that the pandemic is to be comprehended in the fluctuating ratios between the known and the unknown, between the existing conditions and the changing quantities. This humility is proper to science.

The course of the pandemic is a matter of relative speeds and relations between speeds. The speeds of the viral infection are already multiple in accordance with the *flight transformations* available to it, which we must understand in the way that Elias Canetti (2012a [1960]) taught us: "It is to avoid [extinction] that, in whatever shape offers, everything living flees" (p. 348).

Canetti found that flight transformations have their twin principles in fear and food. Most often, we dwell selectively on his theory of flight commands determined according to the principle of fear but neglect his reflections on feeding. In *Crowds and Power*, he had also presented the hand as the locus of *the food principle* for men. The human is a fragile animal; between its mouth and food there is a yawning *interval* which can only be traversed by human hands: "It is the quiet, prolonged activities of the hand which have created the only world in which we care to live" (Canetti, 2012a [1960], p. 213).

With hands we eat as well as feed, and we strive to build the technologies and institutions so as to exceed the speed of famines and epidemics. Today, it is the hands of the doctors and health workers that traverse the living, the dead, and all the medical techniques which strive to prevent the piles of corpses described by Thucydides.

Now, a virus itself is a type of mobile genetic element that becomes active and virulent only when transposed in its host environments. It is its proliferation within, for instance, the human animal under certain circumstances that results in an epidemic. This is where the principles and the relative speeds of human flight transformations become salient. In an epidemic, it is a question of the interacting relative speeds, say of the sprayed and deposited viral droplets and global contact and transport systems of humans. The dispensers of health and public order, too, measure their plans in terms of the relative speeds – of setting up hospitals, acquiring medical equipment, testing, developing a vaccine and harvesting, trading and distributing food.

Speed is the measure of things turning with respect to each other. At a certain point doctors understood that the high rate of oxygen flow through intubation might not suit all patients, as their lungs are diseased to differing extents. As one doctor said, in some cases: "It's like using a Ferrari to go to the shop next door, you press on the accelerator and you smash the window" (Aloisi et al., 2020).

The probing art of the clinical practitioner is to find such proportional articulations.

The world itself, which today connects everyone and everything in unprecedented ways, is an immense and dynamic arrangement of co-articulated components, that is, regularities within which things interact at determinate speeds. This arrangement only ever had degrees of proportional articulation – say between demand and supply, lending and profiting; while its other components abided in a disproportion whose span is not yet revealed – unemployed populations, stateless refugees, nuclear wastes, un-operationalized technologies and also the yet to be imagined possibilities of politics that would respond to the problems of everyone in the world. Added to this arrangement is the virus as a new speeding component. The lockdowns seek to decelerate the flight of the virus. This is, however, also accelerating the decay of the present world system of exchanges that sustain humans (though not well). The pandemic has occasioned certain exchanges of speeds such that this world machine is seizing up like an overheated engine. What care does this moment need?

Many today cling to hypophysical habits of thought by equating care with reparation (Mohan & Dwivedi, 2019). Heidegger (1975) sought to displace this equation by translating the surviving fragment of Anaximander. It was thought to say: "according to necessity; for they must pay penalty and be judged for their injustice" (p. 39), but in Heidegger's philosophizing translation, it said: "along the lines of usage; for they let order and thereby also reck [care] belong to one another (in the surmounting of) disorder" (p. 47).

In this way, the fragment offered the 20th-century thinker the plain-speaking riddle of the being of all things. For him, the being of all things came about in successive, ordered interrelations, in a such a way that each order (or arrangement) depended on and yet differed from the previous one. He found that none of the orders disclose, and therefore all of them hide, *the dispensing of these orderings*. Hence, Heidegger (1975) thought of being as an illegible destiny because what bound the successive orderings as one history was not revealed. And further he considered this "already forgone destiny of Being's oblivion" (p. 51) as the very history of the West; its dawn was in Anaximander's intimations of this destined oblivion, and its twilight was the accomplished oblivion of the 20th century with its technological establishment of man as master of earth (Heidegger, 1975, p. 57).

But this 21st-century viral pandemic has criticalized our world. That is, it has shown the limits of some of the world's components as well as the unrealized powers of certain others. Let us entertain for a while a playful analogy between a fragment of a lost text and a virus. The philosophical fragment is a *mobile thinkable element*, and Heidegger had handled it as such. Today, let us assay another transposition of the Anaximander fragment. That is, we can make its intimations of "usage," "order" and "reck" once again mobile, but this time, without seeking the restoration of an original Greek destining.

Destiny and destination, which have the sense of coming to a stance, share the speculative root –*sta*, "to stand, make or be firm." The human animal came newly stumbling into a world that was not the bucolia of the middle panel of Bosch's *The Garden of Earthly Delights*. Rather, it was a vast unwelcome in which one learnt, with the help of each other's sustaining hands, to walk, to build and to suffer wrecks whether by storms or by one's bad arrangements. One did not seek to reconstruct either a first space of arrival or the last collapsed edifice. One sought to make a new arrangement, which would reserve its future ruin as a surprise. We speak today of sustainability as though the world's destiny – whether betrayed by technological man or fulfilled by abstinent man – were there awaiting revival. We speak of apocalypse today as though a destiny of decline, whether traced by Adorno or Heidegger, was "forgone." But the proportionally articulated components, which enjoin things into a world, linger only in wait of coming disproportions. They gain new components of relative speeds and their new articulations. Only *a while* separates their stance from their in-destinacy. They compose a more or less temporary arrangement, a world, which is soon vacated for another arrangement, another world. *Then, that place, which lets worlds come and go, is none other than this very world experienced as indestinate.* Forsaken by origin and end.

Our world now relates everyone everywhere in an arrangement of reciprocal, though not equal, interactions – actions across distances, mobile effects. We witness this in the spread of the pandemic as well as in the effects of the lockdowns. This makes us responsible for everyone everywhere. Regionalities cannot isolate themselves from materials, ideas, diseases and news which come from the next city, state, country or continent. Governments rush to ease their ill-planned lockdowns, hoping perhaps to revert to pre-existing global arrangements, but *we* realize that this is a hesitating interregnum of decelerations in order to rearticulate the speeds of the whole world's components. It can be an opportunity to rearrange our presently minimized regularities in order to find new accelerations for *the care of everyone.* Then, we must recognize ourselves *as the world*, and we must call and answer to the world as the world – a democracy of the world.

Instead, we are being called back by regional loyalties in philosophy, politics and care. The theories of "modernity" developed at the beginning of the last century were yearnings against two centuries of industrialization and growth of crowded cities. The theorists proposed that the evil of totalitarianism emerges from the "deracination" of countryfolk and the emergence of floating "masses." The world appeared to them *destined to decline* through an increase of something bad called power. Once again today, we are being told that life flows outside isolation, in human crowds, but at the same time we are quickly checked from flying too far, crossing borders, losing roots, crowding metropoles. And so the flight from the coop ends just inside the barn.

But in the pause of the lockdown, we do imagine other flights. Canetti's analysis of the flight transformations between crowds, packs, herds and institutions shows the polynomia of indestinacy. *Polynomia is the power of the mind to legislate different regularities in the same object.* Among these many types of crowds, Canetti found that the specific formation of fleeing as an unregulated "open crowd" offers the experience of equality and dissolution into non-individuated humanity. Agamben's (2020b) biopolitics seeks this open crowd as the norm of human life. But insensate freedom from ourselves through a lurching mass in intransitive flight is another species of release from life itself. And Canetti knew it to be a rare, fleeting phenomenon. He pointed rather to "the patience of the hands": "words and objects are accordingly emanations and products of a single unified experience: representation by means of the hands. . . . the instruments of these transformations" (Canetti, 2012a [1960], p. 218).

By patience he meant not slowness or stillness but readiness for transformations. Reading Gandhi is the most instructive for us to recognize the false problem of crowd and isolation. He proposed the ideal village life of restriction to a minimality where the human hand would be staid. Canetti intimately knew and shrank from this stasis (Mohan & Dwivedi, 2019) as he recounted experiencing it in his book *The Voices of Marrakesh*: surrounded by clamouring beggars in a cemetery, he says, "I could feel the seduction of having oneself dismembered alive for others" (2012b [1968], p. 50).

Researchers and reporters who reason with the world know that solutions cannot be engineered from outside the conditions, needs and desires in this indestinate world (indeed, the only solution of this kind being proposed now suggests that we should do nothing and "let live" or "let die" in accordance with some invisible destiny). *We today*, however, respond to problems of the *worldwide* exchanges of speeds and regularities, not just those of provinces or nations. Our flight is of collective findings as well as inventions, of preparation as well as the unlooked-for. It is, to retranslate the Anaximander fragment,

> along the lines of indestinacy; for they must exchange arrangements and be re-articulated with one other, coming over stasis.

References

Agamben, G. (2020a, April 23). A question. *Autonomies*. http://autonomies.org/2020/04/giorgio-agamben-a-question/

Agamben, G. (2020b, April 7). Social distancing. *Autonomies*. http://autonomies.org/2020/04/giorgio-agamben-social-distancing/

Aloisi, S., Beasley, D., Borter, G., Escritt, T., & Kelland, K. (2020, April 23). Special report: As virus advances, doctors rethink rush to ventilate. *Reuters*. www.reuters.com/article/us-health-coronavirus-ventilators-specia/special-report-as-virus-advances-doctors-rethink-rush-to-ventilate-idUSKCN2251PE

Canetti, E. (2012a). *Crowds and power* (C. Stewart, Trans.). Continuum. (Original work published 1960)

Canetti, E. (2012b). *The voices of Marrakesh: A record of a visit* (J. A. Underwood, Trans.). Penguin. (Original work published 1968)

Heidegger, M. (1975). *Early Greek thinking* (D. Farell Krell & F. A. Capuzzi, Trans.). Harper Collins.

Mohan, S., & Dwivedi, D. (2019). *Gandhi and philosophy: On theological anti-politics*. Bloomsbury Academic.

Thucydides. (1998). *The Peloponnesian war* (S. Lattimore, Trans.). Hackett. (Original work published 431 BCE)

Part III
Psychoanalysts speak

21 Psychoanalysis, too, will never be the same

Néstor Braunstein
May 1, 2020

This coronavirus pandemic is an historic event with unprecedented features, distinct from the multiple previous episodes of the plague in animals and humans. A pandemic is a disease that attacks all or most of a population, a universal to which there may be exceptions. Conceptually it falls within the discourse of science ("science is an ideology of the suppression of the subject") and that of sociology. In principle, the pandemic should be an avatar that homogenizes its inhabitants: everyone is or can be its victim but, as seen in this case, far from that, the disease highlights the differences of wealth and power, underscores the hegemony of the few over the many and makes evident the latent violence present in the social bond under capitalism. We are not all "in the same boat" as it was originally presumed.

However, the pandemic is not an object of the discourse of psychoanalysis, because the latter does not deal with the "all" (*pan*) nor with groups of population (*demos*), although it does deal with the inevitable repercussions of this jarring avatar of social life. In light of current events, it is clear that, as always, those "many" affected by plague, by war, by fear of the many forms of an apocalyptic future, are distinguished by each one's particular circumstances. The threat that presently weighs on the population can be real and viable, like a nuclear war, or imaginary, like a UFO. In any case it is, and in an exemplary form, a phenomenon of language that can extend to planetary proportions and be the trigger of singular fantasies that are, indeed, objects of psychoanalysis, which in turn raise symptomatic formations and decompensations of structure with alterations in the Borromean chain. Many of these are reinforced by the transformations in the conditions and habits of everyday life in its different spheres (familial, work-related, sexual, etc.). Depending on its structure, every *parlêtre* informed by the disruption resultant of the pandemic witnesses and suffers the activation of primary processes of the unconscious that determine its position in life (subjective position, not nosological) faced with the forced recognition of a threat with ill-defined contours, impossible to ignore, generative of obligatory legal restrictions that involve limitations on the freedom to circulate, travel and get together with others. Life is more than ever subjected to the possibility of death, like in war. The confinement demands a "voluntary servitude" (La Boétie, 2016 [1576]), which most of the population complies with for fear of illness and death.

Under these circumstances, in both our clinical practice and in our reflections, our duty as psychoanalysts is to underscore the necessary distinction between "all" (*pan – demos*) and "each one" of our analysands, affirming the irreducibility of the sociological fact, supported by statistics, to the subjective experience reflected in the *transferential* situation that is characteristic of analytical work.

The coronavirus is a biological fact. Coming from who knows where, this contagious disease is an historical and social event studied by medicine. Information regarding the disease and the diverse approaches to combatting it are the focus of lively political and philosophical debates that absorb the attention of the populace of which few, if any, can escape in this media-saturated world. However, each one, as an individual, as a subject-object of communication and according to his own subjective coordinates, shapes a certain response, non-transferable and singular, that confronts the blind and faceless entity which is the virus lurking from its minuscule invisibility.

It is crucial that we do not confuse psychology (the cognitive-behavioral, the individual and social preconscious) with psychoanalysis, which is immune to calculation and statistics, those most contagious of diseases that are transmitted through the media whenever the conversation turns to the "mental" advantages and disadvantages of life in confinement.

What is specific to the psychoanalytic clinic teaches us that the subject of the unconscious, the *parlêtre*, the entity that comes into being because it speaks and confronts death, is faced with an unusual form of the object *a*, a segment of the real lacking a specular image, that carries with it the *Unheimliche*, an uncanny connotation of the possible imminence of its death and that of others. Around this ungraspable object (namely, the virus), fantasies are organized that combine the two poles of desire (will of power, symptom) and jouissance (eternal return, repetition compulsion), Eros and Thanatos.

Hence, the virus today represents the subordinating sun around which subjects of the *demos* revolve in whimsical orbits, called upon by the media to express themselves in this whirlwind of a prevailing confusion of tongues, where "everybody speaks and screams at each other, but nobody knows anything". So too psychoanalysts: we are witness to these predictable but unexpected forms of *civilization and its malaise*; we are pillars upon which rest all of the fantasies brought to light by our "patients" in session as well as "expert" opinions, including we who are called to give testimonies, to render judgement, to express our prejudice and to manifest other *preconscious formations*.

We may conjecture – and this is another fantasy – that the virus with its unpredictable mutations is here to stay and will change the conditions of life in every corner of the planet. It is an object *a*, aphonic, *infans* and ineffable, that has come to embody the position of both *semblant* and *agent* in a wordless discourse that we have begun to feel and that can be thunderous and deafening.

The outdated Cold War option, "freedom without security or security without freedom", which defined the systems on either side of the Iron Curtain, is now heard applied to the ubiquitous and omnipresent virus qua great inquisitor and interpellant. The bell tolls with aeviternal questions: what can I know? what should I do? what am I allowed to expect or hope for? and ultimately, the fourth one: who are you, *parlêtre*, to formulate these interrogations, who will listen to your replies?

We must respond in and with action. There are no subterfuges or artifices: one is always responsible for one's position as a subject. That relationship with the fantasy, brought to light via the analytic setting, is what summons our presence in so far as our individuality is the social subjectified (Korman, 2020) and in so far as "the unconscious is the political" (Lacan). We are and will be the answers we give. We well know that one's own death does not exist for the unconscious; death is always what happens to the Other, and this *otherness* is indelible and moreover underlines our inescapable responsibility for its life.

Within and through the fantasy, our "attitude towards death" (Freud, 1979a [1915]) is decided. In it is played out our position regarding reality, which for the majority is that of a "naked life" (Benjamin, 1994 [1940]), the life of one who is dead without his murder constituting a crime, that of the *homo sacer* (Agamben, 1998), that of the "human flow" (Wei Wei, 2017).

This is how being exposed and vulnerable and the possibility of facing survival post-contagion become the objects of a *biothanatopolitics*. The virus has exposed the always known precariousness of existence as well as the growing vacillation of institutions, of democracy, of the remnants of freedom, of respect for the fantasy of the other, the inhabitant of manipulated choices in the life of the flock that is the *polis*. The virus today invades the cells of citizens with its burden of fear, anguish, terror, mistrust of the social bond, where the other is a fearsome source of danger. Covid-19 does not multiply like cancerous cells but destroys by infiltrating and disordering the intimate life of the attacked cell – and of the psychic apparatus. Thus, it reaches the neuralgic centers (certainly not neurological) where algorithms govern and make their decisions.

Amid the pandemic, the practice of psychoanalysis faces new horizons and must conform to the virtual nature of sessions in which the analysand or supervisee can say (and we now have experience of this): "I cannot speak about that via Skype or WhatsApp," and where the invocation of the fundamental rule of our practice is of little use. This is not paranoia in as much as analysts and analysands well know that there do indeed exist suspicious persons, "flagged" on Google, that undertake their analyses and their supervisions under the possible gaze, and yet impossible to prove nor to stop, of that Other, the guard or sentinel.

The tentacles reaching out from the "societies of control" (Deleuze, 1990) belong neither to the realm of the imaginary nor the phantasmatic. It is there that lurks the danger for the life of the social and for psychoanalysis beyond the oft-praised advantages of digitalization – in the *bio-psycho-technological* control of the telematic power over the species. Freud (1931 [1930]) wrote, by way of concluding his malaise in civilization,

They (human beings) know this, and hence comes a large part of their current unrest, their unhappiness and their mood of anxiety. And now it is to be expected that the other of the two 'Heavenly Powers', eternal Eros, will make an effort to assert himself in the struggle with his equally immortal adversary. But who can foresee with what success and with what result?

"*Le cadre de la cure*" is shifting directions. This has been transpiring at a rapid pace and in multiple ways for more than half a century with impacts on all the varied processes of psychoanalysis in both intension and extension. In the move from the analytic apparatus to that of screens mediating the psychoanalytic dyad with their corresponding satellite interposition and interference by the big Other, aren't the basic conditions of the clinic transformed? And if so, who can foresee with what success and with what result?"

**Translated from the Spanish by
Florencia Bernthal Raz and
Fernando Castrillón**

References

Agamben, G. (1998). *Homo sacer: Lo que queda de Auschwitz* [*Homo sacer: Sovereign power and bare life*]. Pre-Textos.

Benjamin, W. (1994). Tesis de filosofía de la historia [On the concept of history]. In *Discursos interrumpidos*. Planeta. (Original work published 1940)

Deleuze, G. (1990). Postscriptum sur les sociétés de contrôle [Postscript on the societies of control]. In *Pourparlers* (pp. 274–278). Minuit.

Freud, S. (1931). El malestar en la cultura [Civilization and its discontents]. In *Obras completas* (Vol. XXI, p. 140). Amorrortu. (Original work published 1930)

Freud, S. (1979a). "De guerra y muerte: Temas de actualidad", II: Nuestra actitud ante la muerte [Thoughts for the times on war and death?]. In *Obras completas* (Vol. XIV, p. 290). Amorrortu. (Original work published 1915)

Korman, V. (2020, March). *Usos personales de la topología lacaniana en la clínica* [*Personal uses of Lacanian topology in the clinic*]. Congreso de Lógica y Topología en Psicoanálisis, en prensa.

La Boétie, E. de (2016). *Discours de la servitude volontaire* [*Discourse on voluntary servitude*]. P. B. Payot. (Original work published 1576)

Wei Wei, A. (Dir.). (2017). *The human flow* [Film]. Amazon Studios.

22 Politics of the letter

Screened speech is the foreclosure of the littoral of the letter

René Lew
May 24, 2020

In reference to Néstor Braunstein's "Tampoco el psicoanálisis volverá a ser lo que era" (Psychoanalysis, too, will never be the same)

The "social link" is modified by the SARS-CoV-2 pandemic. This change affects *philia* in all its forms: in the family, in love, at work, between friends, in politics, as well as in psychoanalysis. Indeed, the truthful term "social distancing" has produced its effects, despite efforts to cover up its accuracy by the use of more exact terms such as "physical", indicating a separation of bodies. For, in fact, what has occurred is the disregard of the littoral of bodies, and what prevails is a strictly regulated non-relation.

I have already discussed in this series the anathema cast on the littoral of the letter. I have also discussed the real of this anathema in terms of the littoral of bodies – offering or sacrifice.

But a form of relation persists: mediated (telephone, internet, etc.). Sometimes regrettably. What is feared is direct contact, which disappears – for a time – for the sake of distancing. This means that another littoral is introduced, and that the letter immediately acquires another utility which will become clearer in the future. I believe that from now on what predominates is the political function of the letter – as I hinted by pointing out the prevalence of non-relation over relation (sexual, signifying. . .), and this is brought about by organising the characteristics found in abundance on the littoral: each subject bears their mark in his body, to the detriment of non-mediated relations.

In analysis the transference was affected – because there was no direct contact. Many analysts replaced it with a substitute such as the internet or the telephone, or suspended analysis altogether (as I chose to do during the confinement).

Does this mean that object *a* – with its own "littoral character" between abjection and *agalma* – is transformed in this situation?

The pandemic is capitalism; capitalism is pandemic

Must psychoanalysis follow this trend of banishing the littoral of the letter (this banishment is even (if I give the psychiatric terminology a psychoanalytic orientation) a perverse *Shonung* – in that it is perverse to banish the existential essence of all subjectivation of significance? When death (whatever the cause: viral pandemic or "socially" determined death in the camps, and I am not confusing the two registers) is presented as taking precedence over the death drive, it is the littoral of life (referred to death, which precedes it, in the interlacing of sex and death) which suffers, because it is a littoral between life and death.[1]

Death, in writing, in the written account of life and death, is political, as political as the letter itself.[2] The spread of SARS-CoV-2 is itself political: boundless capitalism, involving all human activities, is in no way ecological and destroys the planet, or at least the ecological balance necessary to preserve life (that of plants and animals – and soon, we have reason to fear, that of humanity). The Covid-19 pandemic reveals political (as well as social and health-related) failures and the ecological devastation wrought by capitalism. Indeed, the political governs the life and death of people, their diseases, as well as their subsistence and reproduction, which are tied to material production founded on the workforce (WF) and – if we refer to workforce schemas – on phallic jouissance (PJ):

$$(WF \rightarrow (WF \rightarrow CG))$$
And $(PJ \rightarrow (PJ \rightarrow SE\star))$.
$\star$Lacan's "surplus-enjoyment".

All this cannot be strictly biological; it is clearly a biopolitical question.

Indeed, the widest spread is that of the capitalist system; its destruction of the ecological balance appears to have produced the SARS-CoV-2 virus. We can say that the capitalist system produced Covid-19. There is no need for the virus to have escaped from a laboratory. While the pandemic is imperialistic like capitalism, the virus is the real concretisation of a signifier. The world over, deaths result from the destruction of health systems, which facilitated the capitalist and financial takeover of capital gain (CG) redistributed socially through state budgets or the budgets of health insurance and social security systems (where they exist), created through hard struggle against those who possess the wealth and their boundless desire for profit.

Thus, the relation to death has changed: it is now much more socialised than in the past. Specifically, death is repressed, mourning is resented by the families of the dead – and death no longer enters the domain of life. Mourning rituals are disappearing. Funeral feasts in France are an example. At the same time, the right to be sad is being taken away, because it interferes with the socially organised desire which sustains an equally boundless rapid consumption bulimia. Small shops are disappearing, to be replaced by department stores. Only some food stores remain, but many traditional French deli shops have been converted into Chinese fast-food shops. Fortunately, there are still bakeries, although those willing to perpetuate this hard craft are mostly from the Maghreb. In the cities (nowhere else), all that is left are convenience-type stores, bakeries first and then clothing stores, with banks figuring third in order of importance. Sadness becomes "depression" (a term also used in political economy, come to think of it!) and calls for the use of medication.

The 35,000 deaths caused by the Hong Kong influenza in France were less distressing than the 28,215 deaths caused by Covid-19 (French Ministry of Health) at the time of this writing. Yet 1969 – after the May 1968 events in France – was already the present era. We can certainly place the start of our era 50 years back.

The problem is the desire to know (if the information is exact and properly transmitted) in *real time* everything that happens in the world. The media has aired 24 hours a day what is said (everything?) about this single subject of the pandemic, every day for at least three months. And everyone (!) can keep score of the dead everywhere in the world. (Could this be a remnant of recursion, although such self-reference is censured?)

The signifier takes on a different character

The signifier appears simply as the real:

- Out of reach of the letter (even when protective restrictions, no doubt justified, are issued in writing); and
- Carrying an affective charge of anxiety, in addition to factual information about what is being done and what should be done to treat as well as to prevent, of course.

For instance, there is the guilt felt by children, universally designated as "healthy carriers", who therefore feel responsible for the possible death of adults around them, first and foremost the elderly. A good thing for healthcare spending, no doubt. The children's guilt makes them reluctant to return to school, for fear that they might cause the death of their teachers.

The absence, in contexts other than the "household" (INSEE-style terminology), of directly addressed speech modifies the signifier (S_2) by modifying the meaning (S_1) carried by speech, presumably used to convey the truth. This differs greatly from many false narratives produced nowadays to pacify.

The confinement provided no protection beyond the period when it was maintained: 4% of the French population (based on a Pasteur Institute survey) and up to 10% of the population in the Paris region were infected by the SARS-CoV-2 virus. This falls well short of the 60% "herd immunity" needed statistically to stop the progression of the pandemic. Thus, at the end of the confinement, things are as before for most people. At best, the lockdown made it possible to relieve the burden on hospitals. But – let us stay hopeful – there is no sign of a "new wave" of infections. So far, so good; but we have more to learn about the dynamics of coronavirus infections.

The silence of public authorities about many collective and social aspects of the pandemic is not comparable to silence in psychoanalysis. The latter only acquires meaning in the session, with both people present, not over the telephone. This is so because, over the telephone, any real communication (in which speech conveys truth) is itself cut (crosswise) by mechanical distancing; it loses some of its ambiguity (which promotes significant poetic production), revealing only the realistic aspects of things, with their phantasmatic substrate left untouched. This is why I find that telephone or video analytic sessions – or in the absence of the voice, the use of written discourse – acquire ipso facto a "merely" psychotherapeutic character.

A real void (Lacan's forclusive hole in the real, more than object lack, which remains ambiguous) takes the place of the symbolic void. For instance, the breath of the analysand (or the analyst) is heard differently than in a session "in person". The impossible character of the non-relation dominates, without the intervention of the third person who transmits speech directly. This speech is productive thanks to the littoral transcription of non-relation (each letter/character is distinct from another, with no possible connection between them except vocal or written expression) in the signifying relation.

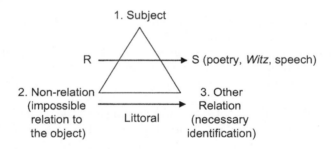

Third-person schema

In the non-relation (without the "poetic" production of speech), the impossible traps the subject in a psychosis-precipitating sideration – in which, knowingly or unknowingly, each person found himself thrown during the confinement. The problem this created was generalised (we might say social) anxiety, although it did not affect everyone. Such a change in the status of anxiety underscores the altered function attributed to Freudian representation (even significance): its metonymic transformation into a communicable virus, replacing speech (which needs no media, and not being a medium itself – no offense to Lacan – is truly existential), embodies the real where the symbolic is demolished by politico-economic agencies, and more generally, we might say, by the pan-liberal civilisation.

But not everyone is overwhelmed by anxiety; everyone is not equally vulnerable to this foreclusion. The problem is that the spread of SARS-CoV-2 – which is not an object a^3 – introduces a transformation of objects *a*: they are no longer actual lacks apprehended as objects, or understood transactions (including intrinsically, and this is an amazing feat, since the apprehension of extensions of meaning is by definition extrinsic), but only substitutes for objects *a*, grafted in stunted form on the autism displayed by our leaders. The duality of the object, at once the object of desire and its cause (given the impredicative definition of the predicative quality of objects), is restrained by the impossibility of establishing a dialectical relation between the intention of speech and an extensional world. Speech becomes misleading; it is used as an instrument of enslavement (this is not new) and no longer requires – as it would if it were truthful – its immeasurable transcription in this object *a*, which is both cause and rejection of desire.

In my opinion, psychoanalysts must refuse *screens*, because their name spells out the truth very clearly: machines put up a screen, and speech (from the Divine Word to the human word) does not accept being machined, that is (in Victor Tausk's terms) becoming an influencing machine. The politics of all the proponents of neoliberalism, including Macron, have led to this health crisis, with its lack of hospital beds and ventilators; with masks, white coats, hairnets and gloves in such short supply that they were unavailable to the general public; and drugs proven effective – at least when symptoms are detected early – that were (and are) prohibited and cannot be prescribed by general practitioners.

Questions raised by the pandemic[4]

Two questions come to mind, one concerning Covid-19 and the other psychoanalysis.

I ask myself, concerning the pandemic and its status (its "value") as a signifier, but also concerning capitalism: how can we all be (this is also "pandemic") so indifferent to the news about the deaths caused by *hunger* in the world: 25,000 a DAY (latest figures from the Food and Agriculture Organization and other United Nations agencies). This is the daily equivalent of all the deaths from Covid-19 in France over a period of two (let's say three) months.

As for analysis conducted using a screen, I do not think it is some sort of "fate" of the modern world. I think it is a choice and a kind of deviation comparable to Lacan's observations in the 1950s concerning certain aspects of the *American way of life*.

We cannot hide behind Covid-19 to justify the perpetuation of this practice in the future, because there are consequences. Analysts must be careful not to betray the fundamental principles of psychoanalysis. Indeed, we must not slip from a justified practice (admitting that it is) in certain conditions – those of the pandemic – at an exceptional time, into a practice that becomes "normalised" without any underlying justification.

Translated from the French
by Agnès Jacob

Notes

1 See part 4 of this series.
2 Lew, R. (2015). *Politique du corps et de l'écriture*. Lysimaque.
3 In fact, an object *a*, a fortiori surplus-enjoyment, cannot be transmitted as such (it is impossible to let someone else enjoy it, or to lose it to someone else who takes it away). In order to be transmitted, it must first be transcribed as a (unary) signifier, and it was for this very reason that the pass was introduced.
4 My reformulation of remarks made by Ana-Claudia Delgado.

23 *Hestiation*

Our life after coronavirus

Sergio Benvenuto
March 20, 2020

1

For some time I'd been meaning to sketch a text of a prophetic nature on the way we will be living in the not too distant future: most of the activities we still conduct in public today will be carried out from home. I'd even found a "scientific" name for this mutation of our lifestyles, naturally taken from ancient Greek: *hestiation*, from Hestia, the goddess of the hearth and the center of home (the Roman Vesta). But the measures imposed to curb the spread of coronavirus have suddenly made my "futuristic" hypotheses as topical as ever. I think that even after we've defeated Covid-19 (if we ever manage to), our life will never be quite the same again. Processes that were already gradually taking place will see a huge acceleration. The larger companies have established the strategy of *working remotely* (a work arrangement Italy was remarkably behind on). The emergency will teach companies and businesses, even smaller ones, that letting their employees telework from home will be far more cost-effective for them and less stressful for their workers. The rite of clocking in and out of an office will be considered terribly old-fashioned: *time spent at the workplace* will no longer count. What will be important is *what you produce at home or elsewhere*. A generalization of piecework. One result will be fewer traffic jams at peak hours. And employees will no longer be forced to see colleagues they loathe every single weekday. Everyone can plough through their work when and where they want, even late at night.

This *hestiation* will also take place in new domains like video teaching, both cost-effective and time-saving: no commuting, lower school maintenance, and wider job opportunities with no need to live where one works.

This revolution has gone hand in hand with online shopping (like Amazon) and entertainment (like Netflix), with products and movies provided directly to our homes, with the delivery person being the new proletariat.

(The gradual disappearance of movie theatres is agonizing for a cinephile like me, knowing I'll never be able to again experience my charming strolls as a young man from one cinema to the other in Paris viewing old, rare, exotic and precious films in small but plush spaces shared with a few spectators, all of us transported to an at once collective and very private world.)

Paradoxically, there will be a resurgence of live theatre, which gives us direct contact with *something happening here and now in a place where we can be physically present*. This close, tangible relationship with artists, the possibility to talk or reach out to them, may even change the architecture of theatres: the stage will be more and more set within the parterre, as it was, in a way, in ancient Greek theatres.

Equally agonizing – for people of my venerable age – will be the disappearance of all those small charming sundry shops, typical of Italy even today. The historical centres of big European cities would gleam with the discreet twinkle of their eye-catching signs and merchandise displayed in display cases – all to be replaced by restaurants, cafés, pubs and nightclubs.

Personal ownership of cars will become increasingly rare. One flies to a destination and hires a car. The narcissistic possession of a car – wasting our time with road taxes, vehicle tests, insurance, maintenance and repairs – is already being replaced by car sharing. Owning a car will increasingly be considered a luxury, as it was 100 years ago.

2

In a world where home will be at once the place where we live, work and entertain ourselves, domestic architecture will change radically. The home will tend to be a closed, autarchic and independent universe: parents working from different rooms, children being video-taught at the dining table and religious services available online, just as Pope Francis is doing now because of the quarantine.

I can already hear the various Cassandras who will read the end of community life in this withdrawal to a miserable domestic ghetto. But in fact, this hestiasized society will take on different forms. We will meet other people not because *we're forced* to (at the office, cinema, shops) but because *we want to*. Personal meetings will be more and more like recreational events and not part of our daily routine. Social life will be more and more a theatre and less and less a workshop. I am not saying all of this to exalt this new form of life – on the contrary, for some (the elderly) it will be awful, while for others (the young) it will simply be their reality, their natural landscape, the way life has always been.

Cities will be full of restaurants and cafés instead of stores and cinemas, because "going out" is something telematics cannot replace. We will need a fresh, different setting in which to meet up with others and *touch* them.

In other words, if I were to give advice to an ambitious young man or woman who wanted to start up a business, I'd suggest opening a restaurant, a bar, a delivery service, a car-sharing company, a theatre or an assistance service.

3

I mentioned the deep aversion this envisioned (but highly likely) world evokes, especially among the not so young.

For example, most schoolteachers abhor video teaching, saying that physical contact with students is essential and so on. The truth is simply that it's hard for everyone to deeply change their habits, even for those supporting Bernie Sanders or Yanis Varoufakis. It's a little like the passage from silent cinema to talkies: many stars of silent movies disappeared because they couldn't adapt to talking, and even the great Chaplin showed initial resistance before eventually doing so. Rudolph Arnheim, one of the greatest cinema theorists, wrote a book (*Cinema as Art*) wherein he argued that silent black and white cinema was true art, while spoken (and in particular color) cinema was only commercial entertainment.

Every technological innovation provokes an initial aversion, and as Roy Lewis argued:

> Even in Paleolithic times there must have been aging conservatives who execrated the innovative frenzies of those who tried to rebel against nature by inventing fire, arrows, spears, matrimony, exploration and such devilish ideas. "We would have been better off remaining trees!" they would probably say when the world around them had already changed, yet again.

Perhaps my easy, though at times painful, acceptance of technological innovation – despite having been born in faraway 1948 – derives from the fact that when I was sick at home one time (I must have been around five), my philosopher father, "the professor", didn't buy me a book but comics, which my mother believed to be damaging. The fact that a philosophy professor would give me comics was for me the definitive authorization not only to accept the new media, but also to harbour a certain respect for popular art forms – or "commercial", as they're referred to derogatively. I would also add the influence of my paternal grandfather, a Neapolitan lawyer, a socialist since his early youth, who died in his late eighties in the 1970s. In his affable, elegant style, he would say:

> I cannot understand my peers, always nostalgic about the old days, always complaining about the present, saying that young people today are too rude. . . . I personally think life is far better today, even in Naples, than it was when I was young. You no longer see slobbering old men, cripples, hunchbacks, barefoot street urchins.

At that time, being a socialist, left-wing, meant being fond of (even technological) progress, while being left-wing today means complaining that the world is getting worse, that everything is becoming degraded – or, as we Italians love to say, "we were better off when we were worse off".

When television first appeared, people started saying that the waves emitted from the TV were bad for our eyes, especially for children (the younger generations always seem to become the elective victims of technological innovations). (But today we spend the best part of the day in front of computers, and no specialist says it damages our eyes.) Whereas now concerns centre around the violence TV exposes our youth to (as if the *Iliad* were not full of violence). Even a renowned philosopher like Karl Popper wrote an anathema, *Television: A Bad Teacher*, in which he denounced TV addiction as a corruptor of youth (the same accusation levelled against Socrates, which led to his being condemned by the people of Athens to be executed by drinking hemlock). This attack against television is absurd; it's like saying that print is a public danger because books like Hitler's *Mein Kampf* have been published. The worst uses of a new medium are invoked to try to discredit that medium as a whole.

So when computers and the internet came along, it was also feared that young people would spend too much time surfing the Web, where they might come across proposals from pedophiles, or more recently, risk becoming *hikiko-mori*, isolating themselves in the company only of the Web. But were things any better when certain young people withdrew to convents or joined the French Foreign Legion?

Not to mention smartphones – heaven forbid! It's being said that "young people are looking at the world through a little rectangle". Old age has only one advantage: it knows that technologies change, but that the conservative answers are always the same. The eternal return of the same old mantra.

4

Finally, I'll dwell on a more specialist issue: the growing tendency to hold psychoanalytic or psychotherapeutic sessions via video. Many important analysts claim that video sessions can never be analytic, backing their claims with excellent theoretical arguments, some taken from a more sophisticated psychoanalytic theory such as that of Lacan. With merely theoretical arguments, that's the point. But the telematics revolution will forge ahead anyway, and more and more analysts will hold sessions via video, Skype, Zoom or Webex. And while video doesn't work with all analysands, the mobility of modern life will end up imposing it – and theory will adapt. After all, Freud had theorized the impossibility of analysing children, psychotics and perverts, and as for group analysis, Freud thought it was unimaginable. And yet while Freud was still alive, his followers (including his daughter) began to analyse children, psychotics, perverts – and the necessities of war led to the discovery of group analysis (Bion's small groups with "impossible" soldiers).

The arguments of analysts who reject video are basically those used by teachers: the physical presence of the analyst is essential to the analytic relationship. Sacred words, but in a world that no longer possesses anything of the sacred, one where everything is fluid, liquid, ever mutating.

I myself have even yielded to video analysis, because more and more patients have become mobile for work reasons. Others want an analysis from abroad, adding linguistic distance to an abysmal geographic one: analysis between an analyst and an analysand, neither of whom is using their mother tongue.

Video seminars and supervisions are also increasingly common, with clinical cases being discussed between analysts. For example, I have supervision sessions with analysts residing at the same time in Novosibirsk (Siberia), Saint Petersburg, Vienna and the United States. Like it or not, this is today's world.

24 The virus and the unconscious

Diary from the quarantine

Sergio Benvenuto
March 29, 2020

Politicians, philosophers, moral thinkers and journalists in Italy are repeating the same concept: "This epidemic is an opportunity to improve ourselves!"

A recurring consolatory idea, believing that if we go through catastrophes, tragedies, wars and calamities, we *will* come out of them improved. Adversity strengthens our character, as the common saying noted. For example, the fact that close contact between people is reduced to a minimum today will make us more eager in the future – they sing – for human contact, sociability, for being-with. Again and again we are told that this extreme privation of physical contact will teach us to relish physical relations once it is all over: we will be much keener to kiss, hug, pat each other on the back, walk arm in arm and so on. This syrupy rhetoric – perhaps a necessary one to console the masses – assumes that painful experience helps us improve. But it is not something we can take for granted. True, there are dramatic moments when entire populations seem to become heroic, like during the bombings of the last world war, when some would sing as they marched down to the shelters.

But does pain really improve everyone? I strongly doubt it.

In the First World War, masses of Germans lost their lives, but 15 years after the end of that war they put Hitler in power and headed straight for an even more devastating war. Nations do not learn from experience. Individuals even less so.

When the catastrophe is over, it is extremely easy to forget. The patriotic effervescence will evaporate sooner or later – and let's hope it does so *after* the end of the epidemic – and we'll go back to our usual vices, to our habitual pettiness. Few will be the wiser beyond the emergency. The masses will go back to being what they always were, moved by the usual, mostly imaginary passions. Certain tragedies can improve some people, true, but they can also make many others worse. Intellectuals, who are paid to think, should eschew the sugary temptation of self-congratulation.

* * *

As every psychoanalyst knows, unconscious beliefs – things we do not know we believe in – are often stronger than conscious ones, those we acquired through enquiry and education. Reactions to the many dangers posed by coronavirus have made one very deep-rooted unconscious conviction in particular stand out: that children are ultimately weak and the elderly strong.

My daughter's boiler breaks. She has no hot water. She calls the plumber, but he hesitates: "I live with my young children", he says with uncertainty. He is scared of infecting them. For him, like for many others, it is kids above all who need to be protected. But we know that children do not normally fall sick if they catch this virus.

I come across constant examples of this misunderstanding. Yet in Italy we are all coronavirus experts now. Millions of us have read an overwhelming amount of information on the epidemic. So we should all know that the median age of those who have died in Italy is 79 and that the younger the person, the less likely they are to fall ill. It seems evident to me that Covid-19 is carrying out a geronticide.

Is it an atavistic, Darwinian reflex that leads us to think small kids are always the most fragile? Perhaps, but I think the reasons behind this misconception are more unspeakable and contorted.

People worry about children and not about the elderly because deep down they hope the elderly will die. "They've played their part", you may hear some say euphemistically. The elderly are a burden to the young, especially in a country like Italy where the share of over-65s is ineluctably on the rise – where, in other words, the perception is that everyone is working to pay old-age pensions to the seniors.

But why then does this epidemic cause so much fear even among those who are nowhere near old age? Because media propaganda (i.e. government propaganda) tirelessly repeats: "Don't think it's only the over-70s who die; lots of younger people fall ill and die!" So we hear interviews with doctors and paramedics giving evidence of this. The fact that Italy's patient zero, Mattia, is only 38, fits this strategy like a glove.

The reason why the state, playing the role of the wise patriarch, tends to scare *everyone* of *any age*, seems to me quite clear: only if all citizens fear for their lives can senior citizens be isolated and spared. Making everyone believe they are at risk keeps people at a distance from the elderly.

★ ★ ★

As soon as people realize Covid-19 is not just a flu, the masses start swarming the supermarkets in panic, especially to buy toilet paper. This happens far less so in Italy, where even a slum has a bidet. But why is toilet paper the first commodity people fear will run out? Because so many think that epidemics are connected above all to uncleanliness, to *impurity* (to filth or sin). And what could be more unclean than our feces? An old theory associates epidemics to a lack of hygiene. During cholera epidemics, people avoided pork in particular, because pigs too are a paradigm of filth.

So, one of the myths thriving on our smartphones is that the coronavirus is essentially transmitted through the soles of our shoes. So, before walking into our houses we should take them off and leave them outside our door, because the virus allegedly survives on the pavement for hours. Here too the connection between the filth on the streets and contagion seems far-fetched. Instead, fewer imagine that the most probable vector of virus transmission is through a lover's kiss, a fraternal handshake, a perfectly clean drinking glass shared with a child.

★ ★ ★

What disturbs many is the fact that during an epidemic, what really counts are the statistics, and many detest statistics. Yet it is the statistics that *tell us how things really stand*. Now, the most important piece of data by which to evaluate the impact of Covid-19 in various parts of the world is not the simple reliance on absolute numbers but rather the comparison of how many died as a consequence of the common flu in previous years – and this is *a statistic that we can hardly find*. For example, some point out to me in terror that in Lazio (the region where I live), just over 100 people have so far died as a consequence of Covid-19. But as I try to explain, in order to make a real assessment we would need to compare this with the mortality rate in Lazio at around the same time last year. And in fact, we discovered that in my region there was not an increase in deaths linked to the flu but a decrease! This line of reasoning, however, is immediately unpopular: I am accused of underestimating the epidemic. I try to explain that only such statistical comparisons can give us the differential dimension and hence the real extent of the epidemic.

For example, today (July 30) I consult the right statistics: the number of deaths caused by the coronavirus per one million inhabitants. The most impacted countries are Belgium (848), the UK (677), Spain (608) and Italy (581). But everybody talks about US (10th with 465) and Brazil (12th with 424).

Many do not like numbers because they are "inhuman" – but often it is precisely the rejection of numbers that creates countless inhuman catastrophes.

★ ★ ★

In the early days of the lockdown in particular, people longed to turn the mandatory seclusion into a patriotic celebration: Italian flags at windows, people on their balconies shouting "Hurrah for Italy!" or singing the national anthem. I have always found patriotism unbearable, but in this case I didn't mind: the country is at war against the virus and finding a unifying signifier, Italy, in a state of belligerency is inevitable.

But had the lockdown been imposed simultaneously throughout the European Union, would we have heard shouts of "Hurrah for Europe!"? I very much doubt it. There is no patriotic identification with Europe in Italy. We attack European leaders and we consider them nothing but dull bureaucrats: how could they not be, when no Italian feels first and foremost European? If one fails to personify an enthusing signifier, one can be nothing but dull and bureaucratic.

★ ★ ★

Services considered to be essential and thus available during the quarantine include tobacconists and perfumeries (which also sell cosmetics and body care items). In other words, the state recognizes the consumption of tobacco (as of alcohol) as a legitimate peremptory addiction.

Perfumes are also essential, particularly in times of humiliating reclusion: they are the most basic gift, in particular for women, just like flowers – and I do wonder why the latter have not been taken into consideration, too, as basic affective necessities. Florists should be allowed to stay open. A few authentic, non-utilitarian gifts should be possible: a perfume, a bunch of flowers. They represent the beautiful nothingness that dissolves in no time and that confirms, paraphrasing Lacan, that love is giving the other what one does not have.

The emergency has revealed the essentiality of what we never thought as such. The TV connection at my house stopped working, but with remarkable efficiency the pay TV quickly sent a technician in a face mask to fix the problem. TV and the internet, which so many philosophers have attacked as modes of alienation, have proved to be basic necessities: the bread and wine satisfying the hunger and thirst for life.

★ ★ ★

Newspapers are also considered essential services, and vendors can stay open, but don't people just read the newspaper online nowadays? Don't we get all the information we need from the Web? Yes, but older people are still attached to the rite of leafing through a printed daily newspaper. Newsstands are open to comfort the elderly, the part of the population that is most authentically at risk.

★ ★ ★

Some friends say to me: "We envy you, because you've got a dog!" Walking a dog, presumably to allow it to pee and poop, counts as a valid reason for being out. If you take a child for a walk, however, that could be a problem. In fact, a child can be extremely contagious while people think that a dog cannot infect anyone. Some say that dogs have replaced children for those who do not have them, but nowadays dogs have become more reliable children than kids themselves.

A meme gone *viral* (how appropriate that such an adjective should have been in use for quite some time now) on social media reads something like: "Dogs are under extreme stress. They go from one 'walker' to another" and don't know what to pee anymore", imagining the scrutiny of a superego police officer following you and asking sourly: "So, why isn't your dog urinating?"

* * *

Stendhal, who said he actually felt Italian, wrote that Italians are "cynical", that they are such an individualistic and disobedient people. And this is also the opinion Italians have of themselves. This is why there is general astonishment at how the Italians are obeying the stringent regulations issued by the government. Seventy percent agree with the measures; many would like even stricter ones. Why so little "populist" moaning?

The reason for this general obedience is because the quarantine affects everyone, including the rich and powerful. And everyone is exposed to infection, including the rich and powerful. There is no room, in other words, for social envy, for resentment against those who have more. The fact that several politicians have tested positive makes them seem closer to us, more "human".

* * *

There is a lot of talk about if "indispensable necessities" includes seeing lovers, boyfriends or girlfriends. "Staying home" means staying with whomever you live. But what about partners who do not live with you? For many, quarantine also involves sexual abstinence.

A woman takes a taxi to see her lover who lives alone but who also has a regular girlfriend he does not live with. If the police were to stop her, she would use the excuse that she's going to ask for a loan, which is actually true: having had to shut down her business activity, she's in need of money. But a Prussian-like police officer could easily object: "Why don't you have the money wired to your bank account online?" Because a "need" can always be confuted and we all feel like potential offenders.

* * *

Many people today are suspended between several love relationships and various "couples". It is unclear who their real wives or husbands are, their girlfriends or boyfriends, their lovers, or whether there's a "couple" at all. *Where* and *with whom* one has decided to spend this interminable quarantine is a like a divine judgment: THE PERSON CHOSEN is one's authentic significant other. If the person chosen is one's father, mother or aunt – well, this reveals the deep truth about who is our *partner*. If one has decided to spend the quarantine alone, it is because ultimately one's significant other is oneself.

* * *

The pandemic is a breeding ground for urban legends, better known today as fake news. Every epidemic manufactures its plague-spreaders. Blaming a virus as such is not enough; there must be a human guilt too. For some time Trump (it is unclear whether because he's too canny or too stupid; sometimes the two qualities go hand in hand) has been placing the entire blame of the epidemic on the Chinese, referring to it as "the Chinese virus" and purporting himself as the saviour from the yellow peril. Back home there are rumours of dark political and military manoeuvres: a fake theory is circulating that claims that the Yankees are in Europe mobilizing for a war against Russia and that US soldiers are vaccinated against Covid-19 (America has the vaccine but pretends it does not) – but I will stop here with regard to these delusions.

It is quite chilling that it is not only the humble, ignorant or naïve who act as megaphones for these paranoiac rumours, but also even medical doctors, biologists, intellectuals, psychoanalysts and so on.

When we meet, my family doctor makes strange allusions to something or other, but in this case I'm not eager to wring out anything from her about their meaning, given that she would love nothing more than having them wrung out of her. Sometimes the *They* are shrouded in mist, almost unpronounceable like the character of "The Unnamed" in Manzoni's *The Betrothed*, a novel with a famous description of the plague in Milan in 1630. *They* fluctuate through the cracks of conversation with cues like "*not surprisingly* this epidemic . . .", "*somebody* knows . . .", "*behind* it all . . .". It's like in paranoid delusions, which sometimes begin with an imprecise nebulous widespread perplexity and then take on the more specific unequivocal traits of *that particular* persecutor, with a name and surname, whether near or far. Collective paranoias – which are the daily bread of politics, social beliefs and most of what we believe we know – are perhaps a key to understanding individual paranoias, and not vice versa, as is commonly believed: paranoiacs absorb discourses; they provisionally condense them according to their individual leanings. They are mouthpieces for enunciations that pierce through them. And they are not always mere relays: sometimes they create out of whole cloth. But they create something meant to be said to other voices.

* * *

We have heard that some 200 people died in Iran because, terrified by the epidemic, they drank methanol. Alcoholic drinks are prohibited in Iran, so all that was available to them was surgical spirit. Would they have done the same if a bottle of vodka had been available to them?

Something similar happened during the prison riots that occurred in Italy after family visits were suspended due to the virus. Several inmates died after invading the pharmacies and randomly guzzling medications as a preventive cure or overdosing on methadone. It is as if a medication as such had a universal therapeutic potential regardless of the illness for which it was designed – a little like those who travel to Lourdes for *any ailment*.

These Iranians drank something sinful according to the Muslim religion. In other words, in this case medication works as a *pharmakon*, a term which in Ancient Greek meant both medicine and poison. The Iranians, with a dizzying association, came to the conclusion that something banned as a moral poison, namely alcohol, could in that case work as a panacea, a panpharmakon. During a medical "state of exception", as a last resort the evil substance is overturned into something beneficial.

This reminds me of something my maternal grandmother did in 1958, when Italy was hit by a polio epidemic that mainly affected children. I was ten years old, and one evening I thought I felt ill – or perhaps the distress of the epidemic had given me a metaphorical sickness. My parents wanted to call the doctor. My grandmother, who lived with us, ran into the kitchen and came back with a great big glass of red wine to offer me. A rare scene, because my grandmother was a teetotaler and disapproved of the fact that my father had already initiated me into the pleasures of wine as part of the virile education he wanted to confer upon me. In short, my virtuous granny was bringing me a nefarious liquid, which I gulped down thinking she possessed a virological knowledge.

Why such a risqué gesture from my grandmother? What strange metonymies led her to think that a glass of wine was a lifesaver? Like for the Iranians, a logic of signifier reversal was at work: in a state of exception, poison becomes a medication. But perhaps, deep down, the idea of offering a dying boy a forbidden pleasure he is not usually granted was also at play in the same way that someone walking to the gallows was classically offered a glass of champagne. It is as if the secret dream of those Iranians had always been to knock back a bottle of wine, and perhaps this was also my grandmother's secret wish: now, in the face of death, satisfying a forbidden pleasure becomes ipso facto a remedy for death.

25 The talking cure by phone during the lockdown

Monique Lauret
May 25, 2020

The brutal announcement of the closure of all public places and the general lockdown declared by the French government on the evening of Saturday, March 14, 2020, as a response to the Covid-19 pandemic threw the population into anxiety, panic, isolation, disarray and (for some) panic, all overnight. This announcement marked not a transition but a break. Analysts and psychoanalysts found themselves in an unprecedented situation and had to find ways to continue their analytical work, despite this rupture imposed from outside, this collective trauma that has already created Post-Traumatic Stress Disorder (PTSD) in some and will keep on doing so. Shock waves from this trauma are likely to be felt for a shorter or longer period of time. The collective trauma that the explosion of the AZF factory represented for the city of Toulouse in 2001 manifested itself in my clinic for several years. The real happens without warning and devastates the fragments of humanity that its sweeps away along its path.

Psychoanalysis demands the presence of the analyst's body and that of the person in pain who comes asking for less pain. Life is unequal, as is one's own innate psychic force. Some people will have more or less chaotic journeys, most often made up of bruised childhoods, unspeakable repressed suffering, transgenerational traumas that inscribe themselves in the body and in the lives of their descendants the symptoms of the cruelty they have suffered. Psychoanalysis deciphers the figure of destiny, making it less dramatic. Psychoanalysis is a long inner journey that allows, through the roads opened by the work of the cure towards the depths of one's unconscious, to reweave the links of life, of one's desire and of one's word internally and to be born at last as a subject.

"Analytical sessions on the phone are not analysis" was the answer of some colleagues caught in the dogmatic certainties of their knowledge. The framework of the cure defined by Freud is of capital importance to establish the transference and to help the unconscious open up. But this framework must be flexible under extreme conditions; adapting the framework for difficult adolescents – so-called limit states – is a common practice nowadays. During the Second World War, when London was bombed, Melanie Klein continued the cure of little Dick by taking refuge in Pitlochry, in the heart of the mountains of Scotland. Most psychoanalysts agreed to the possibility of continuing the sessions on the phone with patients who were already invested in the process and for whom the transference was already established. It was an initiative taken by those who supported their desire in a singular way. Ethics is one of the fundamental values of psychoanalysis. Ethics consists in a "judgment on our action" (Lacan, 1986, p. 359), as Lacan recalled, proposing an ethics of modern psychoanalysis built on a principle derived from Antigone's 'inhumanity': don't give in to your desire. An ethic of psychoanalysis not at the service of goods but at the service of the tragic experience of life. The desire on which Antigone did not give in was to bury the corpse of her brother Polynices with dignity, to preserve his memory and keep his body from the dogs. Leaving open the choice for patients to pursue their cure by telephone was an ethical position supported by most professionals who did not give in to their desire. The physical containment is not a containment of speech. The analyst's desire is a central question. Lacan posited it as the pivotal point of transference, the 'pure body' of analysis, an essential device for the good development of the cure: "it is what is at the heart of the response that the analyst must give to satisfy the power of transference" (Lacan, 2001, p. 451). A corporeal presence maintained by the tenuous link of the voice was possible, because one's voice is part of oneself; it is being manifested. "Because it links man to language, the voice is the dimension of the signifying chain" (Rabinovitch, 1999, p. 19), writes Solal Rabinovitch, also showing the duplicity of the voice, both signifying and sexual. The voice is an object that detaches itself from the body, originating in the Other (*Autre*); it detaches itself from speech. Analytical listening is also beyond dreams, lapses, fantasies, about the sound materiality of language, this level of signifier that can be revealed, pointed out by the analyst in the equivocation of a word to the insistent homophony it conjures. The poet precedes the analyst on the path to truth, as Freud pointed out. He brings us this 'other side of language' where the sound materiality of words dominates over their meaning, this other side which is the realm of the unconscious.

Most of my patients have wished to continue the work they had started months or years ago in this way, by means of the telephone whose wires transmit from the transmitter to the receiver the word of someone, with all the emotional charge associated with it: the affects, the anxieties, the fears, the emotions of a word addressed to the Other (*Autre*) at the end of the phone. What the message, whether true or ambiguous, aims at is the presence of the other as an absolute Other. "It is essentially this unknown in the Other's otherness that characterizes the relationship of speech at the level where it is spoken to the Other" (Lacan, 1981, p. 48), says Lacan. Discourse essentially aims at being. What surprised me in the first weeks was the new depth of speech, of a true speech, the authenticity of the presence to oneself and to the Other. We shared the same ordeal, the same real-life experience, made up of uncertainty and the presence of death at an uncertain yet certain point in our country's history. Some analytical cures have made considerable leaps forward. This time of deprivation imposed by the lockdown drastically reduced social time, time shared with others, family and friends. An imposed reduction, making do with the little, the almost nothing, the void that echoes in the very name ('co-vid'), but which has at the same time opened up the time of the intimate, inner time, the time for oneself, to think about one's life, one's history, the space left for thought if the anguish is not too invasive. The ability to contain anguish varies from one individual to another. Many people discovered this open time with happiness, those who were running after time, had no time for anything, were running away from their own lives. Winnicott spoke of the ability to 'be alone', the ability, once the anguish of separation is overcome, to be able to 'be with' oneself in times of assumed loneliness. Loneliness is not the isolation felt by the sick and elderly who were condemned to die alone without the accompaniment of love.

Loneliness is also silence, an empty space to be apprehended, to be explored, without the need to have recourse to another helper. Victor Hugo, who experienced great moments of loneliness and isolation in his life, talked of "the great teaching of bitter loneliness". Intimacy opens up the possibility of 'being near', as close as possible to oneself, and perchance discovering oneself as Other. The dimension of intimacy belongs to the human being, to the subject of subjective division. It is an inner space that we can inhabit, visit, expand at our ease. It is a place from which we can come and go freely, take refuge, and re-read the psychic movements of our lives under a different light. It is also the place of resistance in extreme conditions. The Jewish author Etty Hillesum (2008) drew her strength from this in an act of clear-sighted lucidity despite the extreme dehumanizing conditions of the concentration camps. Deported and murdered in Auschwitz in 1943, she had previously recorded in her diary two years of reflections and intimate thoughts about her experience. The Nazis were well aware of this space of inner freedom which they tried to break by all means, even going so far as to prevent prisoners from dreaming. The lockdown would act almost like a Taoist method, reduction as a negative method until one lets go in non-action, or *wúwèi* (无为) in Chinese: the natural power of the natural course of things that can let things happen otherwise. It is this positive path that has allowed some analysts to seize this moment to enlarge their psychic time, their logical time necessary to the understanding of their unconscious desires, of deep psychic movements and their integration. In his seminar *The Ethics of Psychoanalysis*, Jacques Lacan likens sublimation to the Thing (*Chose*), *das Ding*. The artist or the one who works on spiritualizing is the one who, at their own get, gets closest to this central emptiness and to *das Ding*, this place where jouissance is also situated and where sublimation and creativity originate, this central emptiness that the time of reduction has brought closer. Lacan emphasized this emptiness and its appealing effect, an emptiness less to be filled than to be circumvented, in order to surround and veil it.

Another phenomenon that struck me in the early days of the lockdown was the frequency of dreams of loss, death and confinement. Representations more or less fleeting for some, more marked for others whose history has been paved with inner confinement and in the unspoken and non-communication, cutting them off from the world of the living or shutting them in the glass prison of their fantasy. From birth to death, the human being has to deal with loss: a loss that must be accepted, to surpass oneself, to symbolize oneself in order to allow the possibility of transformation and to create something new. Focusing only on the behaviour of individuals by neglecting or denying this question amputates the subject of an essential dimension of life. Our era is marked by the denial of death, and the stacked dead bodies of the current health crisis must not be seen, but the death hidden in the daytime resurfaces in thought and dream imagery. The disregard for the burial ritual noted by Robert Maggiori (2020) bears witness to this contemporary foreclosure of the reality of death and the sacred space that must be attached to it for the respect of human dignity. This 'people of merchandise', as the Yanomami Indians of Amazonia call us, was brutally confronted with the disillusionment of the fantasy of total control and the enigma of life in its most singular dimension.

Our work must be a reflection of the Hippocratic Oath that we have taken: "I will spend my life and practice my art in purity and respect for the laws". This pushes us to scientific and institutional inventiveness. We must invent, always invent, to enable psychoanalysis in motion whose living breath will be able to reanimate mechanized consciences. It is a necessary task, and knowing how to adapt with vivacity and vitality to the rhythm imposed by reality allows us to continue to work with joy and humility towards an ethical practice of psychoanalysis.

References

Hillesum, E. (2008). *Une vie bouleversée, journal 1941–1943*. Le Seuil.
Lacan, J. (1981). *Les psychoses, Le séminaire livre III*. Le Seuil.
Lacan, J. (1986). *L'éthique de la psychanalyse, Le séminaire, livre VII*. Le Seuil.
Lacan, J. (2001). *L'analyste et son deuil, Le transfert, séminaire livre VIII*. Le Seuil.
Maggiori, R. (2020, April 15). *Antivirus philosophique 11*. http://philomonaco.com/2020/04/14/antivirus-philosophique-no11-robert-maggiori/
Rabinovitch, S. (1999). *Les voix*. Eres, Point hors ligne.

26 The truth about coronavirus

Duane Rousselle
March 20, 2020

There are urgent new demands being made to psychoanalysts. They come in
the form of requests for assistance: "help me to wake up from the nightmare
of our current pandemic!" Even Slavoj Žižek has recently confessed that he
thought about going outside to contract the novel coronavirus so that he would
not have to worry about it as a looming threat. This is one way to trick yourself
into gaining the upper hand on the real, but it is unsustainable. Alas, there is no
waking up from the nightmare. To wake up from it can only offer the promise
that the dream will continue in a new form.

The nightmare is a return to the enigma of the drive; it is a return to the
impossibility of making sense of it all. It also opens up the possibility of fabri-
cating new solutions through science – which acts directly within the real – and
through an everyday attitude of hyper-pragmatism. Indeed, we are quickly
approaching the sort of pragmatism that functions in India, from where I am
currently writing. Indians regularly engage in active boundary maintenance
strategies, active negotiations with their environment. And as Max Weber
so forcefully argued many years ago, the Dharmic position on reincarnation
necessitates a fixation on the never-ending life cycle of rebirths, the life which
must finally be put to an end. This is a dream that we have already begun to
dream in America. It is a twenty-first century dream of the real from which
each subject seeks comfort within the dark and chaotic world.

The urgency has now reached a fever pitch while the demand that confronts
us exposes itself more and more in its truth. Amidst all of this, psychoanalysis
becomes a refuge by resisting the tendency to request that the subject isolate
itself further into the real. Who wants to live in a world that forces a choice
between science and the plague? The only choice that the subject sees today is
to turn toward pragmatic science as a response to urgency or else hop around
in a world of constant boundary maintenance to the point of exhaustion or
loneliness. Alas, the nightmare never ends.

Psychoanalysis resists these twin responses and institutes a pact with the
nightmare by putting it to work in the cause of truth. It is not by chance that
the pandemic fits all of the coordinates recently laid out by the World Association of Psychoanalysis, whose last few years of work have witnessed the development of the concepts of urgency, nightmares, panics, the real, enigma and so

on. These are the coordinates for our cold new world and they help us to map the space for a new invention.

Today we must discover a new mode of distanciation from the real without thereby losing our social thread. Psychoanalysis has confronted the enigmatic virus directly as the cornerstone of its discourse and as the thread of its new social bond. Thus, when Freud, on his way to America, said − although there is no evidence to suggest that he actually did say it − "they don't realize we are bringing them the plague", he was, in a way, placing psychoanalysis on the side of the plague. This is already enough to demonstrate that Lacan's rejection of the cure or healthiness as a goal of psychoanalysis is in the spirit of the Freudian discovery. We should be very modest, then, since our goal is not to 'cure' folks from the plague; our goal is rather to find what within the plague offers access to a truth which determines us and might be put to social use.

The real threat today is not coronavirus, necessarily, but the real itself, which gives way to the coronavirus and to all other terrifying and lawless pandemics such as addictions, loneliness, depression, panic attacks and so on. As we struggle to either plug up the real or avoid it (through various techniques of so-called biopolitics, such as temperature scans, masks, self-isolation and so on), we also risk failing to face the structures which gave rise to them. If airports and train stations used to be places of demarcation between one space and another, they have now become fuzzy spaces: the border that separated neurosis from psychosis, like the border that separated the public from the private, has collapsed. And this collapse implies that there will be those who rush to implement new and more cunning ways to manage and control the world.

Capitalism and the pragmatic philosophy underpinning it offer themselves once again as an antidote to chaos: pragmatic science, quick to dip into the real to find a solution, the free-market, and other Christian secular notions of impartial intervention, thrust to the fore while other narratives suggest that coronavirus was a consequence of unchallenged dictatorships. The implication is that capitalism − and the market which pushes practitioners to invent another gadget or pill, another quick fix and so on − is the only sane alternative. This narrative can only think of capitalism and dictatorship, of pragmatism and authoritarianism, which are, in so many ways, two symptomatic responses to the real. But pragmatism was never really a philosophy any more than capitalism was a political-economic system. If the radical philosophers, including Marx and Bakunin, were quick to ask "what about the alternatives?", then it was because they sometimes failed to see that capitalism has assumed the position of 'alternative.' Capitalism is the alternative (to authoritarianism, dogmatism, socialism and so on). Capitalism sells itself not by its explicit convictions nor by its inherent liberties but rather by its 'cash-value' approach to truth (to borrow an expression from the American pragmatists): truth is truthful precisely because it produces an effect that is of some circumstantial value. Capitalism today sustains itself by offering itself as the pragmatic alternative to any sustained conviction.

The trauma of capitalism has its basis within the real. Whether we are subjected to environmental disasters, looming planetary collapse or biological crises, we witness in all cases the never-ending return of the lawless real. This is what Michel Foucault and his followers today (many of whom have had their letters recently published in the *European Journal of Psychoanalysis*) seem to miss: the return to 'bare life' or to 'biopolitics' is a restricted view in that it focuses and foregrounds management techniques without situating these techniques as responses to the new paradigms of jouissance. We must resist the temptation to see biopolitics only as an attempt to manage the real; it consists also of the real intrusions into any such attempt to manage and control it.

This is the engine of politics today; this is the truth of our time.

Index